Boris Mravec

Nervous system

Morphological and functional basis of signaling

Nervous system
Morphological and functional basis of signaling

1st edition

Boris Mravec, MD. PhD.

Professor of Normal and Pathological Physiology
Institute of Physiology, Faculty of Medicine, Comenius University Bratislava, Slovakia
Biomedical Research Center, Institute of Experimental Endocrinology, Slovak Academy of Sciences, Bratislava, Slovakia

© *Boris Mravec, 2024*

The contents of this book may not be reproduced, duplicated, or transmitted without the direct written permission of the author.

Under no circumstances shall the author be held liable or legally responsible for any damages, compensation, or financial loss resulting directly or indirectly from the information contained in this book.

Legal Notice
This book is copyrighted. It is for personal use only. You may not modify, distribute, sell, use, quote, or paraphrase any part of this book or its contents without the permission of the author.

Disclaimer Notice

Please note that the information contained in this book is for educational and entertainment purposes only. Every effort has been made to present accurate, current, reliable, and complete information. No warranties of any kind are expressed or implied. The reader acknowledges that the author is not engaged in rendering legal, financial, medical or professional advice. The content of this book is derived from various sources. Please consult a licensed professional before attempting to implement any of the information contained in this book.

By reading this book, the reader agrees that under no circumstances shall the author be liable for any losses, direct or indirect, incurred as a result of the use of the information contained in this book, including but not limited to errors, omissions, or inaccuracies.

Foreword

The book "*Nervous system: Morphological and functional basis of signaling*", which is primarily intended for students of medicine, natural sciences and related fields, as well as for PhD students in neuroscience, aims to introduce the basic structural and functional characteristics that underlie the generation, transmission and processing of signals in the nervous system. Unless further specification is given in the text, the description of the structures and functions of the components of the nervous system is based on knowledge applicable to the human or mammalian nervous system in general.

The book is designed as an introduction to the study of the nervous system. It describes the structure of the cells forming the central and peripheral nervous system as well as the mechanisms of conversion of external and internal environmental stimuli into electrical excitations, which are subsequently transmitted and processed by neurons. It also describes the chemical principle of signal transmission between neurons and the mechanisms of signal processing at the level of neuronal circuits.

December 2024

Boris Mravec

Content

Part I. Cells of the nervous system   1

1. Neurons.   3
    1.1 The body of a neuron   4
    1.2 Cytoplasm and organelles.   5
        1.2.1 Cell nucleus   5
        1.2.2 Plasma membrane   6
        1.2.3 Ribosomes and endoplasmic reticulum   7
        1.2.4 Golgi apparatus and cisternae close to the plasma membrane   8
        1.2.5 Mitochondria   8
        1.2.6 Lysosomes and peroxisomes.   9
        1.2.7 Cytoskeleton.   9
    1.3 Neuronal processes.   10
        1.3.1 Dendrites.   11
        1.3.2 Axons.   11
        1.3.3 Synapses.   13
    1.4 Types of neurons.   15

2. Paraneurons   17

3. Glia cells   19
    3.1 Astrocytes.   21
    3.2 Oligodendrocytes.   23
    3.3 Microglia   23
    3.4 Schwann and satellite cells   24
    3.5 Glia and sheaths of peripheral nerves and ganglia   24
    3.6 Ependyme.   27

Part II. Electrophysiological characteristics of neurons   29

4. Resting membrane potential and neuronal excitability.   31
    4.1 Resting membrane potential   31
    4.2 Excitability of neurons   35

5. Graded potential and action potential.   37
    5.1 Graded potential.   37
    5.2 Action potential   38

Part III. Signaling-related components of the neuron   41

6. Receptor segment and receptor potential.   43
    6.1 Dendrites and the cell body as a functional unit   43
    6.2 Receptive segment of peripheral sensory and sensory neurons   44

Content

7. Initial and conductive segment **45**
    7.1 Initial segment and integrated potential 45
    7.2 Conducting segment and action potential 45

8. Transduction (synaptic or effector) segment **51**
    8.1 Neuromuscular junction (disc) 51

Part IV. Synaptic transmission and neurotransmission   53

9. Chemical synapses **55**
    9.1 Synthesis of neurotransmitters. 55
    9.2 Storage and release of neurotransmitters. 55
    9.3 Binding of neurotransmitters to receptors 57
    9.4 Removal and recycling of synaptic vesicles and neurotransmitters 59
        9.4.1 Vesicle membranes 59
        9.4.2 Neurotransmitter removal and reuptake 60

10. Neurotransmitters and neuromodulators **61**
    10.1 Effects of neurotransmitters. 61
    10.2 Small molecule neurotransmitters 64
        10.2.1 Excitatory amino acids. 64
        10.2.2 Inhibitory amino acids 66
        10.2.3 Acetylcholine and biogenic amines 67
        10.2.4 Other small molecule neurotransmitters. 74
    10.3 Neuropeptides. 74

11. Electrical synapses. **77**

Part V. Processing of signals in the nervous system   79

12. Neuron as integrator **81**
    12.1 Functions of dendrites 81
    12.2 Spontaneous neuronal activity 83

13. Processing of signal in neural circuits **85**
    13.1 Excitatory neuronal circuits 85
    13.2 The importance of inhibition 85
        13.2.1 Presynaptic inhibition and presynaptic facilitation 86
        13.2.2 Feedback inhibition 86
        13.2.3 Forward inhibition 86
        13.2.4 Lateral inhibition 87
    13.3 Neuronal circuits involving neurons that do not form action potentials   88

List of abbreviations. **89**

References. **91**

Part I. Cells of the nervous system

The tissues of the nervous system consist of several types of cells. Neurons are the cells that are responsible for the generation, processing, and transmission of signals. There are different types of neurons in the nervous system that are interconnected to form neural circuits. There are approximately $100\text{-}200 \times 10^9$ neurons in the human brain. The physiological conditions necessary for neuronal activity are provided by glia cells. These cells ensure the formation of sheaths on neurons and their processes, release growth factors, maintain the homeostasis of the extracellular environment, and remove toxic substances and waste products from neurons. Glia cells are also involved in the formation and maintenance of barriers between neurons and surrounding tissues.

1

Neurons

A neuron is the basic morphological and functional unit of the nervous system. There are more than 50 different types of neurons in the human nervous system, which differ from each other in shape and the functions they provide. Nevertheless, all neurons share common features that distinguish them from the cells of other tissues. An example is the polarization of the neuron cell body and the compartmentalization of functions, which reflects the specialization of neurons for the generation, processing, and transmission of electrical signals. A neuron is made up of multiple structurally and functionally distinct compartments:

- cell body, which represents the genomic and metabolic center of the neuron;
- dendrites, mostly relatively short projections of the neuron body, which represent the main area receiving signals;
- an axon, which runs out from the neuron body, often over a greater distance, and transmits action potentials to presynaptic endings, through which it makes synaptic contacts with other neurons or effector cells (Fig. 1.1)

This arrangement allows neurons to respond to stimuli by generating specific signals (action potentials), transmit them rapidly to other neurons or effector cells and thus influence their activity. The high specialization in signal transmission means that neurons are unable to divide and, if the supply of oxygen and energy substrates is restricted for only a few minutes, they are irreversibly damaged and then die.

Neurons also differ from other cells in that they exhibit an increased capacity for excitability (excitability). Excitability, manifested by rapid changes in the electrical potential of cell membranes, is based on the presence of ion channels and ion pumps in the neuron's plasma membrane.

However, polarization and excitability are not exclusive to neurons. For example, epithelial and non-neuronal secretory cells are also polarized, as they can distinguish between apical and basolateral surfaces, and these two regions differ morphologically and functionally (ontogenetically, both neurons and epithelial cells are derivatives of ectoderm, which explains the presence of polarization in both cell types). In addition, some non-neuronal cells, especially muscle cells, are also excitable.

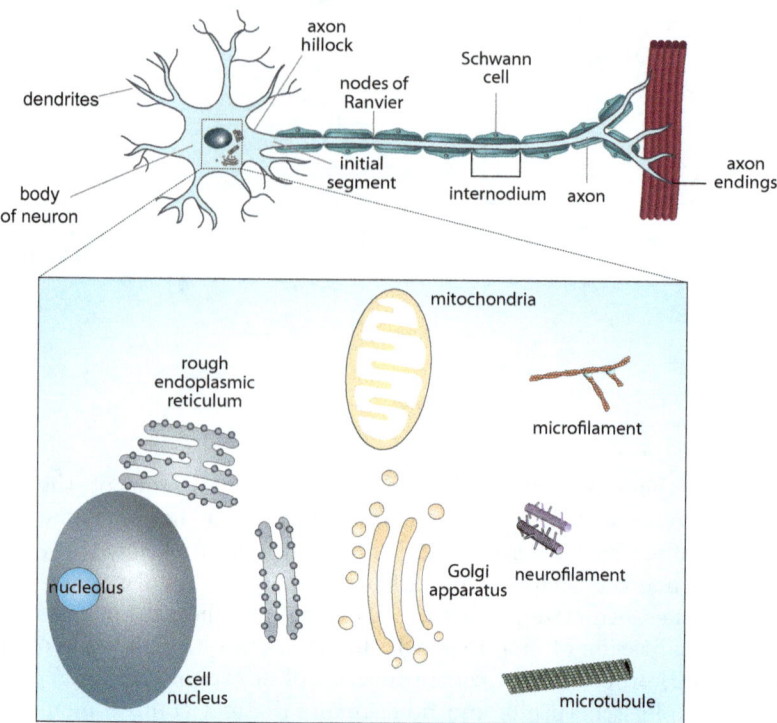

Figure 1.1 Schematic illustration of a neuron and selected organelles. The body of a neuron is mostly composed of several shorter processes, dendrites, and one longer process, the axon. The axon is surrounded by glia cells (Schwann cells). The membranes of adjacent Schwann cells do not completely abut each other, but are separated by nodes of Ranvier. The space between adjacent nodes of Ranvier is referred to as the internodes. The axon can branch; the terminal sections of each branch are referred to as axon terminals (modified according to Coleman, 2005; Bear et al., 2015).

1.1 The body of a neuron

The cell body (soma) is the trophic center of the neuron. It contains the nucleus, which contains DNA, and the apparatus necessary for protein synthesis. Since axons do not undergo proteosynthesis (they do not contain ribosomes or the necessary amount of RNA), these processes are dependent on the proteosynthesis taking place in the body of the neuron. Unlike axons, dendrites contain the necessary apparatus for protein synthesis, which is important for their function, but most of the proteins that are also present in dendrites, are synthesized in the body of the neuron. The body of the neuron contains a whole spectrum of organelles.

1.2 Cytoplasm and organelles

Neurons contain the same intracellular components as cells of other tissues. But there are some specificities that are determined by the basic function of neurons, the transmission of signals.

Like other cells, neurons are separated from their surroundings by a plasma (cell) membrane, which is made up of an asymmetric phospholipid bilayer structure, similar to other biological membranes. The plasma membrane is a hydrophobic barrier that is impermeable to most water-soluble substances. The interior of the neuron is filled by the cytoplasm, which has two basic components, namely the cytosol (which includes the cytoskeleton) and the membranous organelles. The cytosol represents the aqueous phase of the cytoplasm, and only a small number of proteins are freely soluble in this phase, mostly proteins that catalyze various metabolic reactions. A large number of cytosol proteins have general functions common to most neurons, others are specific to particular subtypes of neurons (e.g., enzymes involved in neurotransmitter synthesis and degradation). Several cytosolic proteins are unevenly distributed in neurons, forming clusters, particles, or matrix. Some cytosolic proteins involved in signaling events are concentrated at the periphery of the neuron in the cytoskeletal matrix in close proximity to the plasma membrane.

In addition to the prominent nucleus, the neuron contains a perikaryon, or neuron body, which contains a large number of different organelles. The organelles of neurons include mitochondria, peroxisomes as well as a complex system of tubules, vesicles and cisternae (vacuolar apparatus), which consist of rough and smooth endoplasmic reticulum, Golgi apparatus, secretory vesicles, lysosomes and various transport vesicles that functionally connect the compartments formed by these organelles.

1.2.1 Cell nucleus

The cell nucleus of neurons is large and usually spherical in shape, containing a prominent nucleolus. The cell nucleus is separated from the cytoplasm by a bilayer membrane, also referred to as the nuclear envelope. This membrane contains nuclear pores through which macromolecules synthesized in the cell nucleus are transported into the cytoplasm. In humans, the cell nucleus of neurons, like other somatic human cells, contains 23 pairs of chromosomes made up of deoxyribonucleic acid (DNA) molecules and proteins (additional DNA molecules that code for functional proteins are found in the mitochondria). The outer layer of the nuclear envelope seamlessly transitions and fuses with the membranes of the endoplasmic reticulum. The inner layer of the nuclear envelope membrane contains filaments that bind both to chromatin (a complex of DNA and protein molecules) found in the cell nucleus and to other structures involved in regulating the diameter of the pores in the nuclear envelope membrane.

Chromosomes contain sequences of DNA that are called genes. Genes determine the order of amino acids in polypeptide chains and thus the structure and function of proteins. The transcription of the DNA code into the amino acid sequence of a particular protein is a multi-step process. During gene expression (transcription), specific ribonucleic acid (RNA), also called mediator RNA (mRNA), is produced in the nucleus of the neuron. The newly synthesized mRNA is translocated from the cell nucleus through the nuclear pores into the cytoplasm, where it binds to ribosomes that contain ribosomal RNA (rRNA). mRNA serves as a template that allows the nucleotide sequence of a given gene to be transcribed into the amino acid sequence of a protein. Transfer RNAs (tRNAs) are involved in this process, transferring the activated amino acids to the mRNA, and ensuring that the amino acid chain is gradually built up.

With the exception of a few proteins encoded by DNA found in the mitochondria, all proteins arise from nuclear mRNA in the cytoplasm of the neuron. As in other cells, three basic types of proteins with specific physiological functions are synthesized in neurons:

- Proteins synthesized in the cytosol on free ribosomes and polysomes that remain located in the cytosol of the neuron. These proteins, which are transported by slow axonal transport, include enzymes essential for catalysis of chemical reactions occurring in the cytoplasm.

- Proteins synthesized in the cytosol by free ribosomes and polysomes that are incorporated into the cell nucleus, mitochondria, and peroxisomes. These proteins include enzymes involved in the synthesis of RNA, DNA, transcription factors regulating gene expression and other proteins necessary for the functioning of these organelles. These proteins can be transported by slow axonal transport (also as part of mitochondria).

- Proteins whose synthesis takes place on the membrane system or in the lumen of the endoplasmic reticulum and Golgi apparatus. The synthesized proteins are stored in vesicles that originate in the Golgi apparatus and once released, are transported by rapid axonal transport as part of organelles such as lysosomes, secretory vesicles (containing neurotransmitters), or are transported to the plasma membrane, where they become part of its protein components.

The cell nucleus also contains the nucleolus, which is the structure responsible for the production of rRNA. The nucleolus contains a large number of RNA and protein molecules, and to a lesser extent DNA. The nucleus is a particularly prominent structure in neurons, as neurons are characterized by high peptide and protein biosynthesis activity (neurons are analogous to secretory cells, with the "secreted" molecules being predominantly neurotransmitters).

Cells in the brain express more genes than any other body organ. Of the estimated 19 500 genes, about half are specifically expressed in the tissues of the nervous system.

1.2.2 Plasma membrane

The plasma (cell) membrane is a complex and dynamic structure with a thickness of 8 to 10 nm. Several cellular processes specific to neuronal activity are related to molecular reactions that take place at the plasma membrane. The plasma membrane is a flexible structure consisting of two layers of lipid molecules (phospholipid bilayer) and associated proteins, lipids (cholesterol and glycolipids) and carbohydrates. The surface area of the plasma membrane can only change as a result of the incorporation of another section of the plasma membrane or, conversely, as a result of the detachment of a section of the plasma membrane. In the plasma membrane, lipids are oriented with their hydrophilic (polar) part to the outer layers (intracellular and extracellular) and the hydrophobic (non-polar) parts are oriented to the center of the membrane (bilayer). Thus, the hydrophilic heads are oriented on either side of the membrane opposite the water molecules. Membrane proteins immersed in the lipid bilayer are referred to as integral or intrinsic proteins, with peripheral proteins bound to them. Carbohydrate molecules are found on the outside of the plasma membrane, with those that bind to proteins being part of the glycoproteins and those that bind to lipids being part of the glycolipids. These carbohydrates may be involved in processes related to molecular and cell recognition and also provide cell adhesion. The outer surface of the membrane that interacts with the interstitial space differs both structurally and functionally from the inner surface of the plasma membrane that interacts with the intraneuronal space.

Biological membranes generally exhibit similar functional characteristics:

- prevent the diffusion of water-soluble molecules;
- are selectively permeable to certain ions and molecules, which is provided by specialized pores or channels;
- provide signal transmission through protein receptors that respond to chemical or physical stimuli such as neurotransmitter molecules, hormones, photons, vibrations or pressure.

Thus, the lipid bilayer serves as a barrier that prevents the diffusion of substances and is not freely permeable to ions and molecules. However, it contains proteins that serve as receptors, ion channels and transporters, which determine the selective permeability to certain ions during specific situations.

1.2.3 Ribosomes and endoplasmic reticulum

Neurons synthesize a large number of proteins that are involved in maintaining their integrity and function. Neurons are actually cells that "secrete" neurotransmitters, thus resembling endocrine gland cells. Over the course of 1 to 3 days, they synthesize an amount of proteins equivalent to the total protein content of a neuron. Most of the proteins are carried in the neuron via axonal transport.

Ribosomes are intracellular structures that ensure protein synthesis. They consist of several types of RNA and proteins. Free ribosomes and polysomes are responsible for the synthesis of cytoplasmic and plasma membrane proteins (but only those proteins that are not integrated into the plasma membrane). Individual cisternae of the smooth endoplasmic reticulum are also found in axons and dendrites. The smooth endoplasmic reticulum is an organelle involved in the synthesis of proteins that are secreted from neurons, proteins that form an integral part of the plasma membrane as well as proteins found in lysosomes.

The characteristic organelle of neurons is the Nissl substance. It is formed by basophilic clumps that are found in the neuron body and in dendrites, but

Nissl substance is not present in the axon and axon bump, but it is present in dendrites. Each Nissl body is composed of flattened vesicles, or cisternae of rough (granular) endoplasmic reticulum, on the surface of which are anchored ribosomes protruding into the cytoplasm, free ribosomes, and clusters of ribosomes that form polysomes. In contrast to the rough endoplasmic reticulum of glandular cells, most of the proteins that arise in the rough endoplasmic reticulum of neurons are utilized directly in the neuron, which is determined by the significant functional load on neurons by processes associated with neuronal signaling.

1.2.4 Golgi apparatus and cisternae close to the plasma membrane

The Golgi apparatus is a complex organelle consisting of multiple interconnected flattened cisternae, vesicles and membranous tubules. Various other organelles, including mitochondria, lysosomes and vesicular bodies, are found in close proximity to the Golgi apparatus.

The Golgi apparatus is involved in the formation and modification of protein molecules. Proteins synthesized in the endoplasmic reticulum are translocated through its tubules and vesicles containing newly synthesized proteins are formed by exocytosis of the endoplasmic reticulum membranes. These vesicles are translocated into the Golgi apparatus and subsequently pass through several compartments of the cisternae of this organelle. During passage through the Golgi apparatus compartments, the proteins are modified and sorted before they are translocated into vesicles formed by exocytosis of the membranes of the Golgi apparatus structures. The resulting vesicles contain glycoproteins and secretory products. Glycoproteins are subsequently translocated via plasma transport to different regions of neurons, where they may serve as integral plasma membrane proteins, be released from vesicles into the extracellular space in response to an external signal, or form part of lysosomes, where they function as enzymes. Each vesicle that arises from the membranes of the Golgi apparatus has an "anchor site" on the outer surface by which they bind to the surface of target organelles.

Near the plasma membrane is a system of smooth, flattened cisternae that are tethered to the cell membrane. These cisternae form a second membrane boundary of the cell. These cisternae are thought to be used for the uptake of metabolites.

1.2.5 Mitochondria

Mitochondria are made up of two membranes, with the inner membrane forming cristae that protrude into the inner compartment. Mitochondria are specialized for the production of the energy needed for cell function. Energy, together with water and carbon dioxide, are the products of aerobic cellular respiration and enzymatic activity, with carbohydrates serving as the substrate. The energy released during nutrient oxidation is converted into high-energy phosphate bonds in ATP molecules. Energy in the form of ATP is essential for a large number of cellular processes, including, for example, the maintenance of the activity of ion- and chemical-transporting pumps across the plasma membrane, protein biosynthesis, and axonal transport.

Neurons, unlike most other cell types, do not have stores of glycogen, which is a common source of energy. As a result, their energy processes depend on a constant supply of oxygen and glucose from the circulation. Neurons cannot use lipids as a substrate for anaerobic ATP production. As a consequence of the above limitations, neurons are very sensitive to interruptions in oxygen and glucose supply caused by disruption of neural tissue perfusion.

Mitochondria also contain a small amount of their own mitochondrial DNA (mtDNA), which allows them to synthesize some of the RNA molecules, structural proteins and enzymes needed for their functioning. However, several substances necessary for mitochondrial function originate in the cytoplasm.

1.2.6 Lysosomes and peroxisomes

Lysosomes are membrane-bounded vesicles that serve as an intracellular digestive system. They contain a variety of hydrolytic enzymes that break down and degrade substances produced both in and around the neurons. Hydrolytic enzymes and lysosomal membranes are synthesized in the rough endoplasmic reticulum and are subsequently translocated to the Golgi apparatus where further modification occurs. After exiting the Golgi apparatus, they are transported as vesicles, as primary lysosomes, to the phagosomes, the membrane organelles that contain the waste products of the neuron. Hydrolytic enzymes are released from the primary lysosome into the phagosome to degrade the waste material, and such an organelle is referred to as a secondary lysosome. The material that the lysosomes cleave includes multiple neuronal structures such as receptors and portions of membranes, some of which can be reused. The so-called yellow lipofuscin granules found in older neurons represent signs of wear and tear on these cells and may be formed specifically by insoluble residues in the lysosomes.

Peroxisomes are organelles that have detoxifying functions. They use the enzyme catalase, which hydrolyzes hydrogen peroxide. They are involved in protecting neurons from the toxic effects of hydrogen peroxide.

1.2.7 Cytoskeleton

Adaptation to different shapes, as well as the execution of coordinated and directed movements, depends on a complex intracellular skeleton made up of protein filaments and tubules and their associated proteins, referred to as the cytoskeleton. The cytoskeletal network permeates the body of the neuron as well as its processes, dendrites, and axon. The cytoskeleton is not a fixed structure but undergoes dynamic changes that are particularly evident during the development of the nervous system, neuronal growth and after neuronal damage.

The cytoskeleton consists of multiple filamentous organelles:
- neurotubules (neuronal microtubules), which are approximately 20-25 nm in diameter;
- neurofilament (microfilament) having a diameter of about 10 nm;
- actin microfilaments with a diameter of about 5 nm.

Tubules and filaments contain approximately 25% of all proteins found in a neuron. Neurotubules and neurofilaments are found in all areas filled by cytoplasm. They serve as molecular motors that mediate the transport movement of organelles within the neuron. Actin microfilaments, which are primarily located near the plasma membrane, are significantly involved in the elongation of the growth cones of neurons. Tubules and filaments vary in length but do not themselves reach the length of axons or dendrites. Tubules are structures that exhibit polarity of their end sections. In an axon, the "plus" end of the tubule is oriented toward the axon terminal and the "minus" end is oriented toward the body of the neuron. In dendrites, their polarity is mixed, with about half of the tubules having the "plus" end pointing toward the body of the neuron and the other half having the "minus" end pointing toward the body. Both tubules and filaments are made up of polymers of repeating subunits that are in a dynamic state of constant change, gradually lengthening as well as shortening.

Neurotubules are non-branching cylinders formed by polymers of the tubulin protein. In a neuron, they provide transport of organelles bounded by membranes. While in the body of the neuron they are arranged irregularly in different directions, in axons and dendrites they are arranged longitudinally. Neurofilaments are non-branching cylinders formed by the protein actin and other proteins. They are part of axons but occur in smaller numbers in dendrites. Neurofilament proteins, which are found only in neurons, are part of a group of proteins that includes intermediate filament proteins present in other cell types and a protein found in glia cells (glial fibrillary acidic protein).

A specific property of cytoskeletal components is their ability to transition from a stable state to a state of dynamic structures. In a fully differentiated neuron, the cytoskeleton provides mechanical strength to the neuron and its processes (axons and dendrites) and, via the neurotubules, transport of material from the neuron body to the axon terminals as well as in the reverse direction. The cytoskeleton exhibits high plasticity during neuronal development or during neuronal regeneration after peripheral nerve transection. In these situations, the growth cone uses the cytoskeleton to grow in length, to retract, and to change shape rapidly, serving as a moving sensor.

1.3 Neuronal processes

There is mostly one axon and several dendrites protruding from the body of the neuron. These neuronal processes are referred to as neurites. In some neurons, multiple axons also protrude from the cell body (e.g., Golgi cells in the cerebellum), while in others no axons are present at all (e.g., amacrine cells in the retina). Dendrites are specialized to receive signals; the axon provides transmission of action potentials to other neurons or effector cells. The dense tangle of axons, dendrites, synapses and neuroglia found in the grey matter of the central nervous system (mainly in the cerebral cortex) is referred to as the neuropil.

1.3.1 Dendrites

Dendrites represent the primary receptive segment of neurons. Based on their distance from the neuron body, dendritic areas are divided into proximal and distal. In some neurons, specialized types of dendrites are distinguished. An example is pyramidal cells, which have one large apical dendrite arising from the apex of the neuron, the body of which is pyramid-shaped. In addition, multiple basal dendrites protrude from the basal portion of pyramidal neurons.

Dendrites contain the same cytoplasmic organelles (e.g., Nissl substance, mitochondria) as the neuron body and can therefore be considered an "extension" of the neuron body. Dendrites branch, with the extent of branching reflecting their functional significance. Since dendritic branching is specialized to receive signals from other neurons, the larger the branching, the more signals the neuron can receive. A large number of axon terminals are superimposed on dendrites, and excitatory activity is summed on dendrites, and therefore signal processing occurs in analog mode.

Tiny spiny processes are found on the dendrites of various types of neurons (e.g., on pyramidal neurons of the cerebral cortex). These dendritic spines increase the membrane area of the receptor segment of the neuron. Up to 90% of all excitatory synapses of the central nervous system are located on dendritic spines. Dendritic spines are found in large numbers on neurons of the cerebral cortex, where are involvement in learning and memory processes.

1.3.2 Axons

Axon is specialized in the transmission of signals over long distances. The axon exits the body of the neuron from a structure referred to as the axon hillock in the region of the initial segment and continues for a distance of 1 millimeter to 1 meter, branching at its end into a number of terminal processes that are terminated by a presynaptic ending. The axon hillock, the initial segment and the axon do not contain Nissl substance. The cytoplasm of the axon is referred to as the axoplasm; the plasma membrane of the axon is referred to as the axolemma. The axoplasm contains neurofilaments (microtubules) and mitochondria. Branches of the axon can form two types of extensions containing vesicles with neurotransmitters. Mostly, the branches are terminated by a terminal extension ("knob") that forms a synapse with an adjacent dendrite, cell body or axon of another neuron. In some neurons, extensions called boutons en passage are found along the axons, which do not form classical synapses. The neurotransmitter released from this type of axon "endings" diffuses into the surroundings of these extensions and affects the activity of other neurons, possibly smooth muscle cells or gland cells. A given pattern of axon branching is characteristic of certain types of neurons. Examples are the "basket" plexuses formed by inhibitory interneurons around the bodies of other neurons.

1.3.2.1 Axonal transport

The transport of the entire spectrum of molecules and organelles from the cell body to the processes of the neuron (mainly to the axon terminals) and from the processes to the cell body is provided by axonal transport. In the case of transport from the neuronal body to the processes, it is anterograde or orthograde transport, respectively; in the case of transport from the processes to the neuronal body, it is referred to as retrograde transport. On the basis of speed, a fast transport with a transport rate of 200-400 mm per day and a slow transport with a transport rate of 1-5 mm per day are distinguished. Fast transport can be both anterograde and retrograde, slow transport is only anterograde (Tab. 1.1). Fast anterograde transport is responsible for the transport of mitochondria and smooth endoplasmic reticulum precursors, synaptic vesicles, and parts of the plasma membrane. Rapid retrograde transport involves the transfer of mitochondria, multivesicular bodies (degradative structures) and vesicles containing chemicals such as growth factors that are taken up by nerve endings via receptor-mediated endocytosis.

Axonal transport is provided by neurotubules in conjunction with certain motor proteins that generate the necessary mechanical force to enable movement. Fast transport is generated by the molecular motor proteins kinesin and dynein, which are associated with ATP. These proteins are responsible for generating the mechanical force required for organelle movement by neurotubular axonal transport. ATP molecules are used as an energy source for transport in both directions, with kinesin providing anterograde movement and dynein providing retrograde movement. Meanwhile, each neurotubule contains several "tracks" through which different structures can move. Multiple vesicles may be carried on a single neurotubule, with the speed of movement varying from track to track, or two vesicles may be carried in opposite directions along different tracks of a given neurotube. In addition, during transport, a vesicle may change the neurotubule along which it is transported.

Slow anterograde transport involves the movement of soluble enzymes and components of the cytoskeleton and plasma membrane. Proteins and other substances are transported to restore and maintain the axoplasm of the mature neuron as well as to replenish substances in the growing axon and growing dendrites during neuronal development and regeneration. The protein dynamin is responsible for the slow transport.

Transport system	Transfer speed	Material to be transferred	Molecular engine	Function
Slow	1-5 mm/day	cytoskeletal and cytoplasmic components	dynamin	axon cytoskeleton and axon cytoplasm restoration
Fast anterograde (orthograde)	up to 400 mm/day	organelles bounded by a membrane	kinesin	transfer of material to synaptic endings
Fast retrograde	60 - 100 mm/day	organelles bounded by a membrane	dynein	transfer of material that has been picked up by nerve endings (e.g. growth factors)

Table 1.1 Characteristics of neuronal transport systems (modified according to Steward, 2000; Noback et al., 2005).

1. Neurons

Axonal transport forms the basis for the functionality of the neuron as a whole, as it enables continuous communication between the neuron body and its processes. Through axonal transport, the body of the neuron is "informed" about the metabolic requirements and the state of its most distal sections. In addition, axonal transport ensures the uptake of extracellular substances, such as growth factors, which are transported from the processes to the neuron body, allowing the neuron body to respond to changes in the extracellular environment.

1.3.3 Synapses

A synapse is the point of contact of a neuron with another neuron or of a neuron with an effector cell. There are two basic types of synapses, chemical and electrical. The vast majority of synapses in the human nervous system are chemical synapses. Electrical synapses are present in greater abundance in invertebrates and lower vertebrates; they are present in only small numbers in the mammalian nervous system.

The chemical synapse is formed by the presynaptic nerve ending and the postsynaptic membrane, which are separated by a synaptic cleft. The synaptic cleft, which is approximately 20 nm wide, is flanked by glial cells. The cell membrane of the axon termination at the synapse is referred to as the presynaptic membrane. The membrane of the dendrites, neuron body, or effector cell (e.g., muscle, glandular cell) at the synapse is referred to as the postsynaptic membrane. The region of the postsynaptic membrane directly opposite the presynaptic

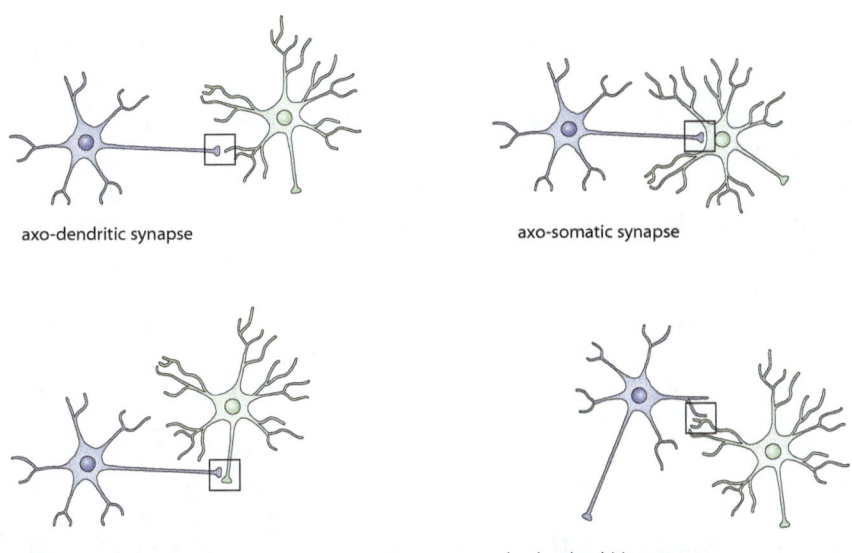

Figure 1.2 Schematic illustration of the types of synaptic connections. Most common are synaptic junctions formed by the axon of one neuron and the dendrite, body, or axon of another neuron. Synapses formed by two dendrites are less numerous in the nervous system (modified according to Feder et al., 2009; Bear et al., 2015).

membrane is referred to as the subsynaptic membrane. In the cytoplasm of the nerve ending, there is an increased accumulation of mitochondria and synaptic vesicles containing neurotransmitters. These organelles are not located close to the subsynaptic membrane. Most neurons contain at least two different types of vesicles, namely small vesicles with a diameter of about 50 nm and large vesicles with a diameter between 70 and 200 nm. Both types of vesicles contain neurotransmitters. Based on morphological characteristics, two basic types of synapses are distinguished:

- asymmetric synapses, which have a dense postsynaptic membrane specialized region, also referred to as postsynaptic densities; presynaptic terminals contain spherical vesicles; asymmetric synapses are found on dendritic spines, dendritic tubes (the portion of dendrites outside the spine processes), and the cell body;
- symmetrical synapses, which have a thin postsynaptic membrane specialization and have flattened vesicles or vesicles of different shapes at the presynaptic ending; symmetrical synapses are found on dendritic tubes, the cell body, and the initial segment of the axon.

On the basis of the structures of the neurons involved in synapse formation, synapses are distinguished formed:

- the axon termination of a neuron and the dendrite of another neuron (axodendritic synapse);
- the axon termination of a neuron and the body of another neuron (axosomatic synapse);
- the axon termination of a neuron and the axon of another neuron (axo-axonal synapse);
- the dendrite of one neuron and the dendrite of another neuron (dendro-dendritic synapse) (Fig. 1.2).

An axon of a single neuron usually makes only a few synapses, but some axons make a large number of synaptic contacts. On the other hand, the dendrites and body of a neuron can make synaptic contacts with many different neurons (sometimes up to 15 000 synapses).

The termination of a nerve fiber on a muscle cell (neuromuscular junction) or on a glandular cell (neuroglandular junction) is similar to synaptic connections between two neurons. The connection between the axon ending and the striated muscle cell is referred to as a neuromuscular disc.

In addition to the common types, less common types of synapses are also present in the nervous system. An example are synapses formed by two dendrites (dendro.dendritic synapse). Such an arrangement is present in the olfactory bulbus, where granule cells that do not have axons are present. Nevertheless, they do form reciprocal dendro-dendritic synapses with the dendrites of mitral cells. In doing so, each dendrite contains a presynaptic region in which there is an accumulation of vesicles, and this region is in close proximity with the postsynaptic membrane of other dendrites. The presynaptic and postsynaptic regions are adjacent to each other, forming reciprocal synapses, forming the basis for locally interacting microcircuits between axonless neurons.

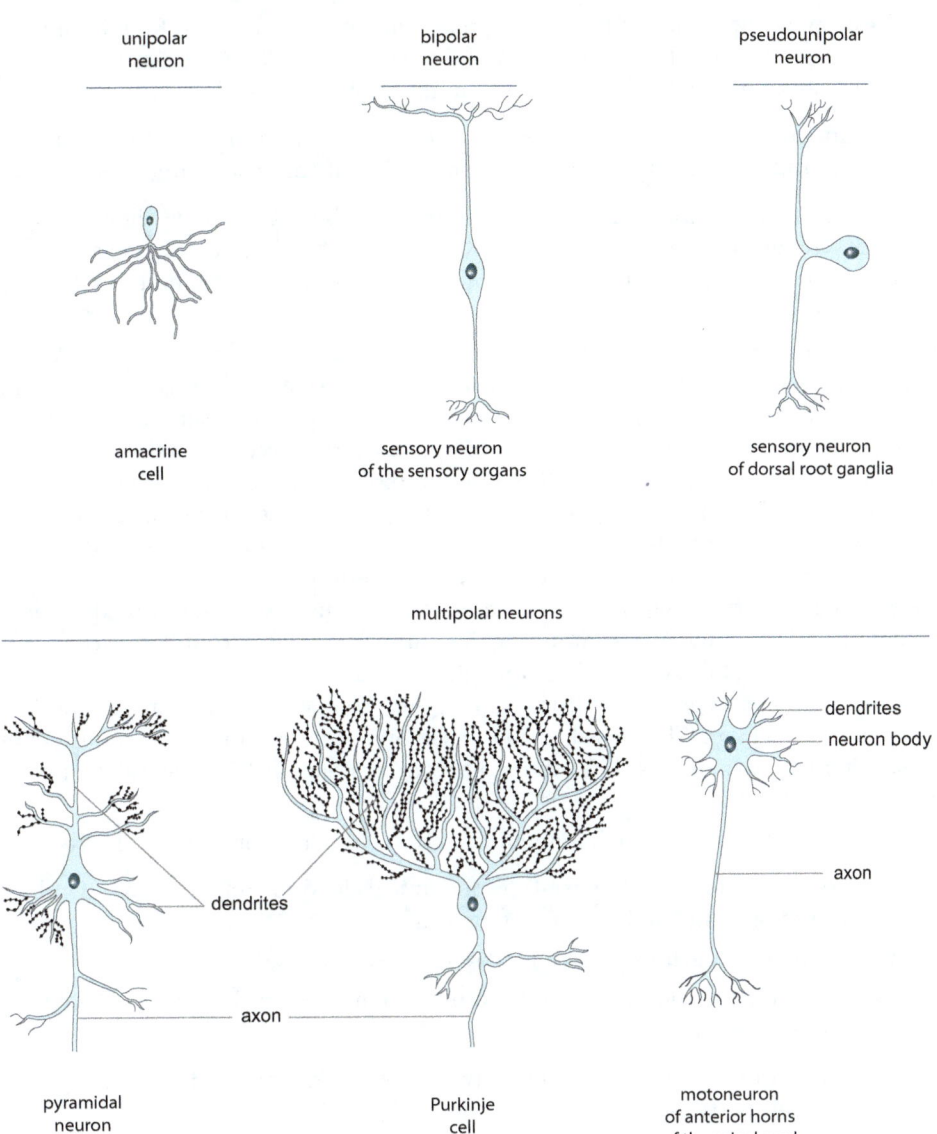

Figure 1.3 Schematic illustration of selected types of neurons that differ in size, shape as well as number and branching of processes. While pseudounipolar neurons are also referred to as afferent neurons, motoneurons are referred to as efferent neurons. Other neurons shown are interneurons (modified according to Badiani et al., 2011; Kiernan and Rajakumar, 2013).

1.4 Types of neurons

Based on morphological and functional characteristics, several types of neurons are distinguished. According to the number of axons and dendrites (collectively referred to as neurites) they are distinguished:

- unipolar neurons, which possess only one neurite; they are found mainly in the ganglia of the dorsal roots of the spinal cord and cranial nerves, they make up about 0.5% of the total number of neurons;

- bipolar neurons, which possess two neurites; located in the retina, inner ear, and taste buds, they make up about 0.05% of the total number of neurons;

- multipolar neurons that possess a large number of neurites; they are found in the autonomic ganglia (about 0.5% of the total number of neurons) and in the brain and spinal cord (about 98.95% of the total number of neurons) (Fig. 1.3).

Unipolar neurons include neurons of the dorsal roots of the spinal cord that have only one process, referred to as a bifurcation, since the process divides into branches. One of these branches projects to the spinal cord, the other branch is formed by a peripherally projecting sensory nerve. However, the cells of the dorsal roots of the spinal cord are actually pseudounipolar, since during development the neuron is bipolar and during maturation the two processes merge into one.

Most neurons in the central nervous system are multipolar and exhibit complex shapes that are characteristic of the neuron type. The aforementioned morphological differences between different types of neurons, caused by differences in dendritic branching and axon branching, are often related to differences in their wiring in neuronal circuits and also in their functions.

The different types of neurons also differ from each other on the basis of dendritic branching. The classification based on the nature of dendritic branching is specific to particular regions of the nervous system. In the cerebral cortex the following distinctions are made:

- star-shaped neurons whose dendrites branch off and branch in all directions;

- pyramidal neurons that contain one apical dendrite and multiple dendrites extending from the base of the neuron.

Based on the length of the axon they are distinguished:

- projection neurons that send axons over a greater distance (called Golgi type I neurons);

- interneurons that send axons only over short distances, in the area where their cell body is also located (called Golgi type II neurons).

Neurons are structurally and functionally differentiated by their location in neural circuits, whereby they are distinguished by:

- primary sensory neurons whose sensory processes are located in peripheral tissues (e.g. skin, retina);

- motor neurons that innervate effector cells (e.g., skeletal or smooth muscle, gland cells);

- interneurons, which make up the majority of neurons in the nervous system and ensure the transmission of signals between other neurons.

Based on the primary neurotransmitter that a given neuron population synthesizes and releases, a whole spectrum of distinct neuron types (e.g., glutamatergic, glycinergic, dopaminergic, serotoninergic).

2

Paraneurons

Paraneurons are endocrine and sensory cells that, although not classified as neurons, share a number of structural, functional and metabolic features with neurons. They can also be referred to as receptor-secretory cells.

Some types of paraneurons are among the cells with neurosecretory function. In response to stimuli acting on receptors on their plasma membrane, these paraneurons release secretory material from granules or vesicles similar to synaptic vesicles. Several of the chemicals released are identical or at least similar to neurotransmitters. Some of the paraneurons whose primary function is the secretion of chemicals are referred to as endocrine cells (e.g. enterochromaffin cells of the enteroendocrine system of the digestive tract). Some paraneurons are sensory or receptor cells, since their primary function is the transduction of signals of certain modalities (e.g., hair cells of the inner ear) (Fig. 2.1).

Examples of paraneurons are:
- rods and cones found in the retina, both cell types having a photosensitive outer segment that represents the modified cilium;
- sensory cells of the olfactory mucosa (neurons of the olfactory nerve); unlike all other neurons, these chemoreceptive cells are exceptional in that they are continuously regenerated by the basal cells of the olfactory mucosa;
- neuroepithelial gustatory sensory cells; these chemoreceptive cells are innervated by afferent fibers of cranial nerves VII, IX and X;
- hair cells in the cochlea, semilunar canals, utriculus and sacculus; these hair mechanoreceptive cells innervate the vestibulocochlear nerve;
- Merkel cells located in the basal layers of the epidermis; these mechanosensitive cells are innervated by somatosensitive nerve fibers;
- the main cells of the carotid bodies, which serve as chemoreceptors that monitor the partial pressure of oxygen, carbon dioxide, and pH of the blood; these cells are innervated by the glossopharyngeal nerve;
- enterochromaffin cells of the enteroendocrine system, a component of the enteric nervous system; these cells synthesize a wide range of gastrointestinal hormones and neuropeptides (e.g., gastrin, secretin, cholecystokinin,

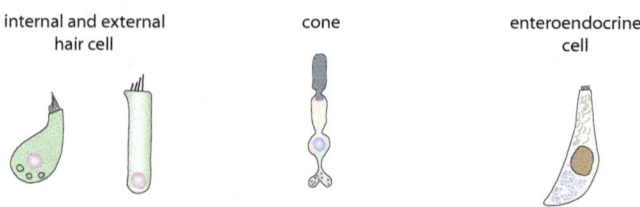

Figure 2.1 Schematic illustration of selected types of paraneurons and their comparison with the enteroendocrine cell. Both paraneurons and enteroendocrine cells are characterized by high secretory activity. While the secretory products of paraneurons mainly serve to communicate with neurons, the secretory products of enteroendocrine cells are of the nature of hormones (modified according to Fujita, 1989; Crosnier et al., 2006; Matthews and Fuchs, 2010).

somatostatin, substance P, and vasoactive intestinal peptide); they are innervated predominantly by parasympathetic nerves, which run mainly in the vagus nerve;

- chromaffin cells of the adrenal medulla, which release epinephrine and, to a lesser extent, norepinephrine into the circulation; they are innervated by sympathetic nerves;
- peptides or amines secreting endocrine cells of the parathyroid glands, adenohypophysis and pancreas.

3

Glia cells

Non-neuronal cells with supporting functions, which are found around the cell bodies of neurons as well as their processes, dendrites and axons, are referred to as glia (neuroglia) and are found in both the central and peripheral nervous system (Fig. 3.1). In the central nervous system, glia cells and neurons are separated from each other by a 10- to 20 nm-wide intercellular space filled with extracellular fluid. This intercellular space constitutes about 15-20% of the total brain volume. In mammals, glia cells are reported to outnumber neurons by a factor of about 10 to 50, depending on the specific region of the central nervous system, with glia making up about half of the total brain volume. But more recent research has shown that in the human brain, the number of neurons is about the same as the number of non-neuronal cells.

Several types of glial cells are distinguished on the basis of function and localization (Tab. 3.1). In the central nervous system, astrocytes (astroglia), oligodendrocytes (oligodendroglia), microglia, and ependymal cells are present. Astroglia and oligodendroglia are also referred to as macroglia. Glial cells in the peripheral nervous system include Schwann cells, which surround nerve fibers, and perineuronal satellite cells, which surround the bodies of neurons. These two cell types, which are functionally difficult to distinguish, are referred to as neurolemmal cells. All glial cells, with the exception of the microglia, arise from the ectoderm during development. Schwann cells and satellite cells originate from the neural crest, which is a derivative of the ectoderm. Microglia cells are predominantly mesodermal in origin. Unlike neurons, glia cells can divide by mitosis throughout the life of an individual.

Originally, neuroglia (nerve glue) cells were thought to have a relatively passive role, providing only limited functions in the central nervous system. It is now clear that the functions of glia are diverse:

- glia form a highly organized "skeleton" that provides the central nervous system with structural support for neurons and neuronal circuits;
- during development, the neuroglia (radial glia) guide migrating neuronal precursors from the neuroepithelium to designated target areas, where definitive patterns of neural circuit arrangement are formed; glia cells also

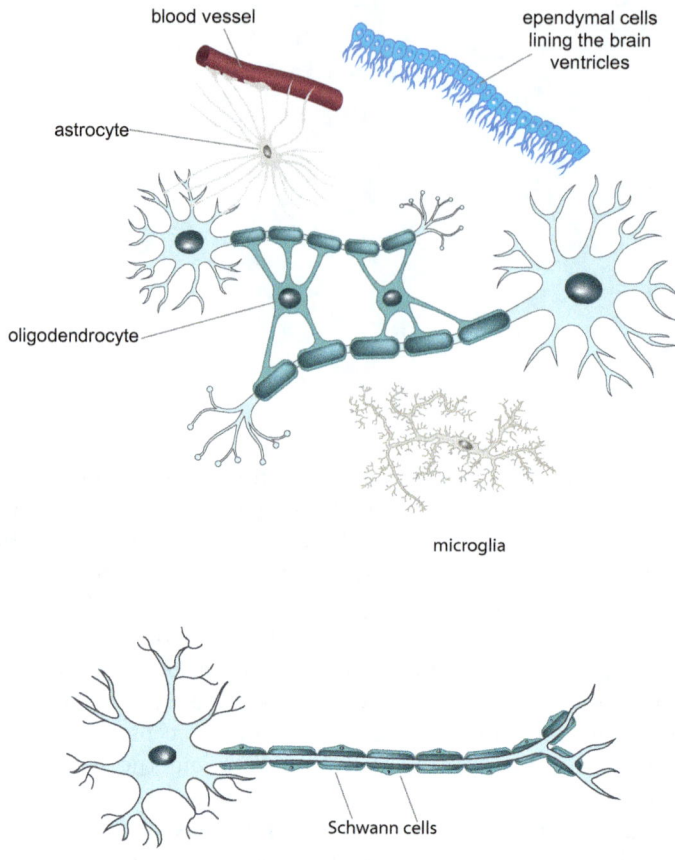

Figure 3.1 Schematic illustration of the different types of glia cells. Astrocyte processes establish contacts with the neuron body and blood vessels, they also delimit synapses. Oligodendrocytes and Schwann cells form the sheaths of axons. Microglia cells are involved in immune functions and debris removal (modified according to Abbott et al., 2006; Ables et al., 2011; Hammer and McPhee, 2018).

determine the direction of axon growth and thus determine the formation of neural pathways;

- glia cells synthetize and release growth factors that prevent neurons from going into apoptosis; growth factors are also required for the processes related to neuronal regeneration and plasticity;
- oligodendrocytes and Schwann cells form myelin, which significantly increases the speed of action potential transmission through axons;
- microglia serve to remove debris (waste material) that is produced after neuronal damage or death and is also involved in immune processes occurring in the central nervous system;

Glial cell type	Location	Characteristic cytological features	Features
Protoplasmic astrocytes	CNS grey matter	star-shaped; long, thin processes that penetrate between neuronal cell bodies, dendrites and synapses; processes forming glia limitans on the surface of the brain and glial feet on blood vessels	spatial damping of fluctuations in ion concentrations (e.g., K+); neurotransmitter uptake; they encapsulate neuronal processes, preventing diffusion of neurotransmitters from one synapse to another
Fibrous astrocytes	CNS white matter	star-shaped; long, thin processes that enter between axons	spatial damping of ion concentration fluctuations
Intrafascicular oligodendrocytes	CNS white matter	send out long processes that form myelin sheaths around the axons of CNS neurons	myelination
Perineuronal oligodendrocytes	CNS grey matter	small cells that are found just adjacent to neuron bodies and dendrites	not obvious
Microglia	grey and white matter CNS	shape resembles perineuronal oligodendrocytes; in response to injury, the processes contract and the cells show phagocytic activity	immune function, phagocytosis
Schwann cells	PNS	cell bodies are found along axons; cells form extensive protrusions of plasma membrane that encircle axons and form myelin sheaths	myelination

Table 3.1 An overview of the different types of glia cells, their localization in the nervous system, their morphological characteristics, and their functions. CNS - central nervous system; PNS - peripheral nervous system (modified according to Steward, 2000).

- astrocytes play an important role in maintaining the homeostasis of the microenvironment formed by the extracellular fluid by regulating the pH and the concentration of potassium ions; they serve as a bridge through which nutrients and oxygen are transported from capillaries to neurons;
- glia cells are involved in the production of cerebrospinal fluid and extracellular fluid that surrounds, nourishes and protects neurons;
- in response to nerve tissue injury, reparative processes are activated, with glia cells proliferating and giving rise to astrocytic scarring.

3.1 Astrocytes

Astroglia form a morphologically and functionally heterogeneous population of cells that surround each neuron of the central nervous system. A distinction is made between protoplasmic astrocytes in the gray matter of the brain near the capillaries and fibrous astrocytes in the white matter. The designation fibrous astrocytes reflects the presence of a large number of glial filaments in these cells, whereas protoplasmic astrocytes contain a smaller number of glial filaments. Other types of astrocytes are Bergmann cells in the cerebellum, Müller cells in the retina, pinealocytes in the pineal gland, and pituicytes located in the posterior lobe of the pituitary gland. These cells contain 8 to 10 nm thick microfilaments consisting of polymerized units formed by glial fibrillary acidic protein, which is their specific biochemical marker.

Astrocytes form a matrix in the brain in which neurons are both located and separated from each other. The cell bodies and processes of the astrocytes are connected by bridging junctions ("gap junctions"), allowing them to function synergistically as a functional syncytium in which ions and molecules are exchanged between astrocytes and between astrocytes and the extracellular fluid.

Like neurons, glial cells also exhibit a negative membrane potential, indicating that their plasma membranes are permeable to potassium ions. However, because the plasma membrane of glia cells contains only a small number of potassium channels, astrocytes are unable to generate action potentials.

Each astrocyte may have several processes that run out into the surroundings, terminating at different parts of the neuron, capillaries, and other structures by extensions referred to as endfeet. These astrocyte endfeet:

- envelop the basement membrane of the capillaries;
- adjacent to the free surface of the cell bodies of neurons and dendrites and enveloping the synapses, thus separating them from each other;
- make contact with the pia mater, thereby forming a pio-glial bounding membrane adjacent to the subarachnoid space;
- make contact with the ependymal cells of the ventricular system.

Almost all substances that enter or exit the central nervous system pass through the cells of the astroglia. Astrocytes carry metabolites, such as glucose, from capillaries to neurons, which they also store. In addition, they uptake potassium ions from the extracellular fluid via potassium channels, in case their extracellular concentration has increased significantly. If there is an excessive rise of potassium ions in certain catchment areas of the extracellular space, astrocytes pick them up and move them via interastrocytic bridging junctions to those areas of the syncytium where the concentration of potassium ions is low (the so-called spatial buffer system). This mechanism prevents the propagation of waves of electrical depression that arise due to the presence of high extracellular potassium ion concentrations, which can induce excessive depolarization of neurons. In situations associated with excessive neuronal activity, they ensure the uptake of glutamate and neurotoxins, which accumulate in the extracellular space and in the synaptic cleft. Thus, astrocytes are involved in the regulation and maintenance of extracellular fluid homeostasis (ionic composition and pH) and in the regulation of glutamate levels in the synaptic cleft, thus providing the necessary prerequisites for the functioning of neurons in the central nervous system. In addition, astrocytes can release several neurotrophic factors (e.g., nerve growth factor and brain growth factor), thereby playing an important role in promoting neuronal survival.

One of the functions of astrocytes is to delimit synapses. Thus, the astrocyte prevents the diffusion of the neurotransmitter outside the synaptic cleft. A single astrocyte encloses several, often thousands of synapses. From the perspective of the astrocyte, the central nervous system is then divided into individual sectors in which synaptic transmission is regulated by a given astrocyte.

By uptake of neurotransmitters (e.g., glutamate, GABA) and synaptic cleft bounding, astrocytes are significantly involved in signaling in the nervous system. Recently, astrocytes have also been shown to be involved in signaling through other mechanisms. For example, astrocytes in the hypothalamus release chemicals known as gliotransmitters, which stimulate receptors for neurotransmitters located at nerve synapses. Thus, glia cells directly regulate synaptic transmission via gliotransmitters, which include taurine, ATP, and D-serine. Vesicles with neurotransmitters are found in astrocytes in various parts of the cell body, from where they can be released into the surrounding.

3.2 Oligodendrocytes

Oligodendrocytes, the glia cells found in the central nervous system, are analogous to the Schwann cells of the peripheral nervous system. Oligodendroglia form and maintain myelin in the central nervous system. Two types of oligodendrocytes are distinguished:
- perineuronal satellite cells, which are closely associated with the neuronal bodies and dendrites found in the gray matter of the brain;
- interfascicular cells that provide myelination of axons in the white matter of the brain.

Numerous processes of individual oligodendrocytes form myelinated internodes on up to 70 axons. The myelin sheath is formed by continuous sheaths forming helical lamellae of the plasma membrane of oligodendrocytes. Myelination of axons begins in the prenatal period and continues in humans until puberty.

3.3 Microglia

Microglia cells, which are of mesodermal origin, enter the central system during the period of vascularization through the pia mater, the wall of the blood vessels, and the choroid body.

Based on functional differences, several types of microglia cells are distinguished:
- resting (inactivated) microglia cells present in the central nervous system during physiological states, also referred to as resident brain macrophages, and this type of microglia can change into the following two types:
- activated or reactive non-phagocytic microglia that are capable of synthesizing cytokines;
- phagocytosing microglia (phagocytes).

Other sources of phagocytosing cells in the central nervous system include monocytes (their precursor cells present in the circulation) as well as meningeal and perivascular cells of the blood vessels of the central nervous system. These cells, when activated by foreign structures and molecules, brain damage, degradation products or inflammation, become 'scavengers', i.e. phagocytes that remove debris from the central nervous system.

The resident microglia are small cells that make up 5 to 10% of all glia cells.

They contain lysosomes and vesicles characteristic of macrophages, only a small amount of endoplasmic reticulum, and few cytoskeletal filaments. They are found as parenchymal microglia in the central nervous system, in the plexus choroideus, and in the circumventricular organs. Microglia may also participate in the formation of neuronal circuits by discarding redundant collateral processes without affecting the viability of the neurons themselves.

Microglia cells are components of the immune system, with activated microglia playing a key role in immune processes occurring in the central nervous system. They are essential components ensuring the interaction between the central nervous system and the peripheral immune system. Microglia engage astrocytes in responses to immune stimuli and are also involved in the synthesis of growth factors and adhesion molecules. These cells can synthesize and release cytokines through which they influence the magnitude of immune or inflammatory responses. Microglia are also involved in processes associated with antigen presentation and thus participate in immune surveillance in the central nervous system. Thus, microglia cells represent dynamic immunocompetent cells that participate in the defense responses taking place in the brain and spinal cord.

3.4 Schwann and satellite cells

The Schwann cells of the peripheral nerves and the perineuronal satellite cells of the sensory and autonomic ganglia of the peripheral nervous system (ganglion glia) represent an analogy to the three basic types of glia cells in the central nervous system (astrocytes, oligodendrocytes, and microglia). Except for differences in location relative to neuronal structures, Schwann cells and satellite cells are almost indistinguishable from each other and are therefore collectively referred to as neurolemmal cells. Like astrocytes, neurolemmal cells both envelop and separate unmyelinated nerve fibers from each other; in addition, they are also found in the interneuronal spaces between neurons. Like oligodendroglia, they form myelin sheaths around the axons of some cell bodies in ganglia. Analogous to microglia, Schwann cells can change into phagocytes in response to nerve injury and in response to inflammation. Unlike glia cells in the central nervous system, Schwann cells secrete extracellular adhesive proteins (collagen, laminin, and fibronectin). These proteins constitute the major component of the basement membrane and extracellular matrix and also form the surface membrane that surrounds the plasma membrane of axon processes. Schwann cells also envelop the axon terminals, which are part of the neuromuscular disc. Glial cells in this area are also referred to as teloglia. Glial cells are also found in the enteric nervous system, which is made up of small ganglia and largely unmyelinated axons. Glia in the enteric nervous system exhibit structural and functional characteristics common to both astrocytes and glia cells of the peripheral nervous system.

3.5 Glia and sheaths of peripheral nerves and ganglia

Peripheral nerves include the cranial nerves and spinal nerves. The peripheral ganglia are clusters of neuronal bodies whose processes are part of the peripheral nerves.

Each nerve consists of three basic components:
- axons;
- Schwann cells (neurolema) and myelin sheaths (interstitial component);
- endoneurium, perineurium and epineurium (connective tissue component) (Fig. 3.2).

The peripheral ganglia also consist of three components:
- bodies of neurons and axons;
- internal satellite cells (interstitial component);
- outer satellite cells (a component of connective tissue).

Schwann cells and the endoneurium provide separation and isolation of individual axons located in peripheral nerves. A group of isolated nerve fibers is joined together to form a bundle that encloses the perineurium. Subsequently, the groups of bundles are joined and delimited by the epineurium. Each of these groups is a continuation of groups of cells found in the peripheral ganglia. The connective tissues contain blood vessels that provide nourishment to the neurons. In addition, these tissues give the nerves both strength and flexibility. This is also due to the abundance of longitudinally arranged collagen fibers, which prevent stretching of the axons, as even a slight stretch affects the transmission of signals in the axons. The flattened cells of the perineurium form a sheath that acts as a physiological barrier that prevents the penetration of chemicals to the axon bundles, thus providing an optimal external environment for axon activity.

The myelin sheath surrounding the axon is formed by multiple continuous helical layers of plasma membrane, with Schwann cells in the peripheral nervous system (oligodendroglia cells in the central nervous system). The myelin sheath

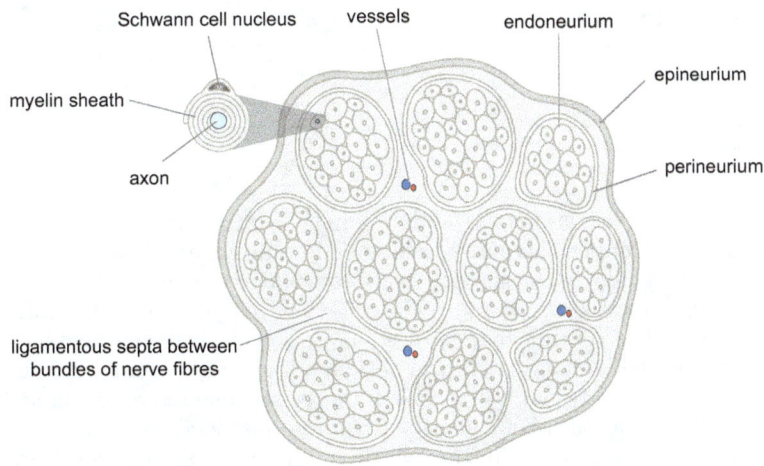

Figure 3.2 Schematic illustration of components of peripheral nerve.

is present in almost all nerve fibers with a diameter of more than 2 μm, whereas fibers with a smaller diameter are unmyelinated.

The myelin sheath is interrupted at regular intervals by Ranvier nodes. The axon sheath between two adjacent Ranvier nodes is formed by a single Schwann cell. The spacing of the Ranvier nodes is proportional to the diameter of the fiber (axon together with its myelin sheath). The thicker the fiber, the greater the distance of the nodes. Fiber diameter and nodes spacing are proportional to the speed of signal transmission (action potentials), with the larger the fiber diameter, the higher the transmission speed.

The Ranvier nodes exhibit some significant structural and functional features:

- axon branching occurs in the areas of Ranvier's nodes;
- the high concentration of mitochondria in the axon cylinder in these areas is conditioned by local high metabolic activity;
- the extracellular fluid is located close to the axon cylinder just in the areas of Ranvier's nodes.

Near the outer surface of each Schwann cell there is a basement membrane, which is synthesized by Schwann cells. It is made up of a homogeneous layer composed of proteins such as type IV collagen and laminin. The basement membrane plays an important role in regenerative processes. The basement membrane is not found around glial cells and neurons of the central nervous system.

While a myelinated nerve fiber is enveloped by its own layer of Schwann cells, in unmyelinated fibers there is one Schwann cell per about 20 axons (Fig. 3.3).

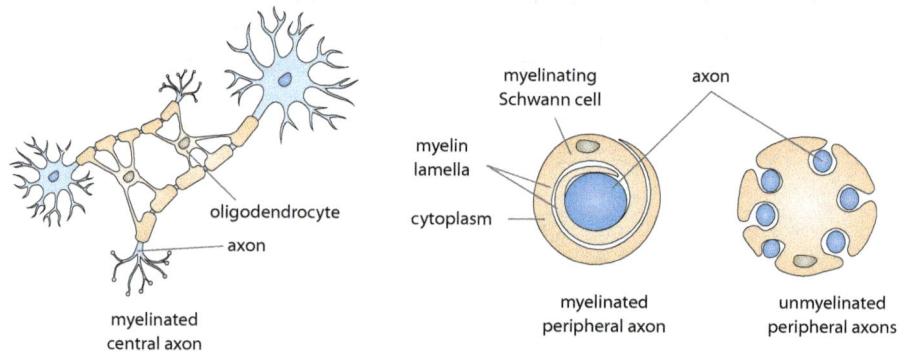

Figure 3.3 Schematic illustration of myelination in the central and peripheral nervous system and comparison of peripheral myelinated and unmyelinated fibers. Myelination is the process whereby glia cells (oligodendrocytes or Schwann cells) surround axons with multiple layers of their membranes. The oligodendrocyte ensures the formation of myelin sheaths in the central nervous system. A single oligodendrocyte forms a large number of internodes on axons. In the peripheral nervous system, Schwann cells provide myelination of axons. One Schwann cell forms only one internode on an axon. The myelin sheath of one peripheral axon is therefore provided by a larger number of Schwann cells. Schwann cells in the peripheral nervous system also surround unmyelinated axons. In this case, a single Schwann cell may surround multiple axons, but it does not form enveloping envelope layers on these axons (modified according to Noback et al., 2005; Mei and Xiong, 2008).

The axons of the olfactory nerve exhibit a specific arrangement, with a single Schwann cell providing the sheaths for several separate axon clusters.

3.6 Ependyme

Ependymal cells are simple cuboidal glia cells that line the central spinal canal and cerebral ventricles. Three basic types of ependymal cells are distinguished:

- Ependymocytes comprise the majority of ependymal cells. Cilia and microvilli are usually found at the apical pole of the cells, which projects toward the ventricular system. The cilia are associated with the basal body, which is fixed in the plasma membrane, while the associated contractile apparatus is responsible for the movement of the cilia. These cells do not form tight junctions with each other and therefore allow free passage of substances between the cerebrospinal fluid and the adjacent neural tissue.

- Tanocytes differ from ependymocytes in having a long basal process. Most of these cells are located at the base of the third ventricle of the brain. Their basal processes penetrate the neuropil and attach to blood vessels and neurons via terminal peduncles. The role of tanocytes is to transport substances between the brain ventricles and blood vessels. An example would be the transport of molecules from the cerebrospinal fluid to hypothalamic neurons involved in the regulation of gonadotropic hormone release from the adenohypophysis.

- Choroidal epithelial cells cover the surface of the plexus chorioideus. At the apical pole of the cells they have microvilli, on the basal surface, which is attached to the basement membrane, there are villi. Adjacent choroidal epithelial cells form tight junctions with each other, thereby preventing the free transfer of plasma proteins into the cerebrospinal fluid. These cells are metabolically active in regulating the chemical composition of the fluid that is secreted from the plexus choroideus into the ventricular system of the brain.

Part II. Electrophysiological characteristics of neurons

Neurons are cells highly specialized for receiving, processing and transmitting signals. The specialization of individual compartments corresponds to this:
- the receptive segment consists of dendrites and the body of the neuron;
- integration of signals is provided by the body of the neuron;
- the segment providing the transmission of signals to other neurons or effector cells is the axon.

The generation, processing and transmission of signals are based on electrochemical principles, and these processes are related to changes in the polarity of neuronal membranes.

4

Resting membrane potential and neuronal excitability

The plasma membrane of neurons separates the extracellular (interstitial) fluid located outside the neuron from the intracellular fluid, i.e. the neuroplasm located inside the neuron. On this membrane, under resting conditions, an electrical charge difference (voltage) is present, which is referred to as the resting potential. This difference in electrical charge between the inner and outer surfaces of the plasma membrane is the result of an uneven distribution of cations and anions, which are present on both sides of the plasma membrane in the form of a thin layer of ions. These ions include potassium ions (K^+) and organic ions (proteins), which are found in higher concentrations in the neuroplasm, i.e. intraneuronally, and sodium ions (Na^+) and chloride ions (Cl^-), which are found in higher concentrations extracellularly in the interstitial fluid surrounding the neurons.

4.1 Resting membrane potential

Several basic electrochemical processes are involved in the generation of the resting potential. Below, hypothetical situations are first presented to describe the emergence of biological membrane polarity, followed by a description of the situation on a real neuronal membrane.

In a hypothetical cell that is separated from its surroundings by a plasma membrane, and which contains no proteins, a potassium salt solution is present (Fig. 4.1). In the cytoplasm of this cell, the potassium salt is dissociated into the cation K^+ (a potassium ion) and the anion A^- (an acidic residue). The same solution is found around the cell, but the concentration of ions is 20-fold lower. Although there is a large concentration gradient between the intracellular and extracellular space, the transfer of K^+ and A^- ions does not occur, as the plasma membrane is impermeable to them because it does not contain ion channels. Under the above conditions, no potential is present between the inner and outer surface of the plasma membrane (voltage difference V = 0 mV), since the ratio of K^+ and A^- on the inner and outer sides of the plasma membrane is 1:1, therefore both solutions are electrically neutral.

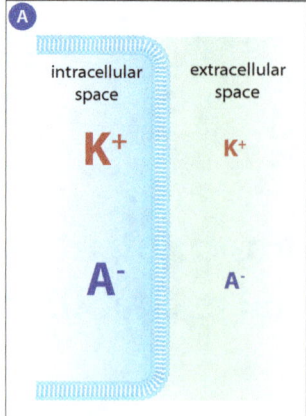 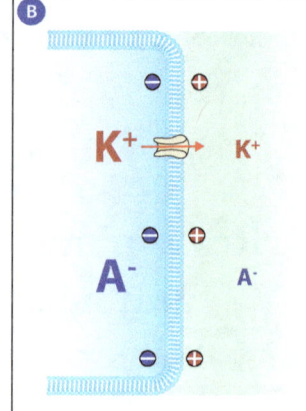 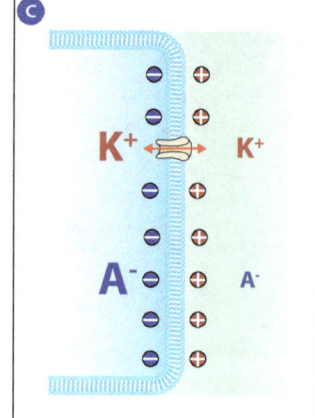

Figure 4.1 Formation of a resting potential at the semipermeable plasma membrane of a hypothetical cell. If the cell membrane is impermeable to cations (K$^+$) and anions (A$^-$), even at different concentrations of these ions in the intracellular and extracellular space, there is no electrical potential difference (A) at the membrane. In the event that channels are present in the membrane to allow the passage of a cation (B), an equilibrium state will gradually develop such that the electrical forces causing the movement of cations into the cell will be in equilibrium with the diffusive forces causing the passage of cations in the direction of their concentration gradient, i.e., out of the cell (C)(modified according to Muchowski and Wacker, 2005; Bear et al., 2015).

The situation in that hypothetical cell will change if channels for K$^+$ ions are present in the plasma membrane (Fig. 4.1). Because the above ion channels are selectively permeable for K$^+$ ions, these ions can freely permeate the plasma membrane, but A$^-$ cannot permeate the plasma membrane. Initially, therefore, K$^+$ ions pass through the membrane to the external environment in the direction of the concentration gradient. As A$^-$ remains inside the cell, a negative electric charge gradually builds up on the inner surface of the membrane, creating a potential difference at the plasma membrane. Gradually, as the internal charge becomes increasingly negative, electrical forces begin to act on the K$^+$ ions, which have a positive charge, in such a way as to induce their passage into the interior of the neuron. Therefore, when a certain potential difference is reached at the plasma membrane, the electric forces causing K$^+$ to move into the cell are in equilibrium with the diffusive forces causing K$^+$ to move out of the cell, in the direction of the concentration gradient. This potential difference is referred to as the ionic resting potential, or resting potential. In the above case, it reaches a value of about -80 mV.

Each ion (e.g., K$^+$, Na$^+$, Cl$^-$) generates its own equilibrium potential in a system of two solutions with different ion concentrations separated by a semipermeable membrane permeable to that ion. The value of the membrane potential can be calculated using physic-chemical laws based on the so-called Nernst equation, which takes into account the charge of the ion, the temperature of the environment

4. Resting membrane potential and neuronal excitability

and the ratio between the concentration of ions between the inner and outer environments separated by a semipermeable membrane.

$$E = \frac{RT}{zF} \ln \frac{[C]_e}{[C]_i}$$

Where:
V (or E) = the difference in electrical potential between the inner and outer space of the neuron, also referred to as the Nernst potential
R = general gas constant
T = absolute temperature (at body temperature its value is 273 + 37 °C)
F = electric charge per gram equivalent of univalent ions (Faraday's constant)
Ci = concentration of ions on the inside of the membrane
Co = concentration of ions on the outside of the membrane

Thus, using this equation, the magnitude of the membrane potential at which a given ion (e.g., K^+) is in equilibrium on each side of the membrane can be determined.

$$E_K = \frac{RT}{zF} \ln \frac{[K^+]_e}{[K^+]_i}$$

$$E_K = \frac{8314,4 \cdot 310,15}{1 \cdot 9,6485 \cdot 10^4} \cdot 2,303 \cdot \log \frac{5,5}{150}$$

$$E_K = 61,5 \cdot \log \frac{5,5}{150} = -88,6 \text{ mV}$$

Thus, the membrane potential of a real neuron depends on the concentration of ions on the outer and inner sides of the plasma membrane, where the concentration of K^+ ions is higher in the neuron and the concentration of Na^+ and Cl^- ions is higher in the extracellular space. Another important factor is the impermeability of the neuron plasma membrane to proteins that have a negative charge and whose concentration in the form of anions is higher in the neuron, since in the extracellular space they are mostly in the form of polymers without a significant electrical charge.

The difference in concentration of individual ions at the plasma membrane of neurons is generated and maintained by a system of membrane ion pumps, referred to as Na^+/K^+-ATPases. This pump is an integral part of membrane proteins and requires energy in the form of ATP for its activity. The Na^+/K^+-ATPase translocates Na^+ ions extracellularly and K^+ ions intracellularly, i.e., against their concentration gradient. The pump transfers 3 Na^+ ions extracellularly and 2 K^+ ions intracellularly in one cycle. This exchange accounts for the fact that the concentration of K^+ is at least 20-fold higher in the neuroplasm than in the interstitial fluid, whereas the concentration of Na^+ is 10-fold and the concentration of Cl^- is 11.5-fold higher in the interstitial fluid than in the neuroplasm (Tab. 4.1). Most neurons do not have a pump for Cl^- ions; their concentration gradient is

Ion	Extraneuronal concentration (nM)	Intraneuronal concentration (nM)	Ratio extra:intra:	V_{ion} (at 37°C)
K^+	5	100	1:20	-88 mV
Na^+	150	15	10:1	62 mV
Ca^{2+}	2	0,0002	10 000:1	123 mV
Cl^-	150	13	11,5:1	-65 mV

Table 4.1 Concentrations of selected ions in the intraneuronal and extraneuronal space and their resting potential (V_{ion}) at the plasma membrane selectively permeable to the ion (modified according to Bear et al., 2015).

determined by passive diffusion of Cl^- ions across the plasma membrane. Since the inner surface of the membrane has a negative charge, a significant electrical force acts to move Cl^- ions into the cell across the concentration gradient. Another ion pump is the Ca^{2+}-pump, which actively transports Ca^{2+} ions from the neuron toward the extracellular space. Intracellular Ca^{2+} binding proteins are also involved in maintaining low intraneuronal Ca^{2+} ion concentrations and moving these ions into organelles such as mitochondria and the endoplasmic reticulum.

The resting potential represents a stable (dynamically equilibrium) state, the maintenance of which requires the energy necessary for the activity of ion pumps creating an ionic gradient on the plasma membrane. During situations when the neuron is at "rest", its membrane potential is the result of a balance between the active Na^+ and K^+ ion transfer provided by the ion pumps and the passive diffusion-mediated ion transfer across the plasma membrane. As the Na^+/K^+-ATPase moves more cations extraneuronally, hyperpolarization of the plasma membrane occurs. The greater the hyperpolarization, the greater the electrochemical forces acting on Na^+ ions (directed intraneuronally) and the smaller the electrochemical forces acting on K^+ ions (directed extraneuronally). The resting state is reached at the plasma membrane when the resting potential reaches such a value that the total passive current directed intraneuronally (movement of electric charge) through the ion channels exactly balances the active current directed extraneuronally, which is formed by the action of the ion pumps. Thus, the resting state is not the result of passive diffusion of ions only, i.e. diffusion in the direction of the concentration gradient, but is dependent on processes requiring energy supply (ion pump activity).

The resting potential of the plasma membrane of neurons is thus the result:

- ion pumps that create a concentration gradient for individual ions;

- plasma membrane impermeability to protein anions;

- by the presence of ion channels, making the plasma membrane selectively permeable for certain ions.

In contrast to the hypothetical cell above, the plasma membrane of the neuron is selectively permeable to multiple ions. The action of ion pumps results in the concentration of K^+ ions being higher in the cytoplasm of the neuron and the concentration of Na^+ ions being higher extraneuronally. If the neuron's plasma membrane were permeable only to K^+ ions, these would permeate outward from the neuron until the resting potential settled at approximately -80 mV. If the neuron's plasma membrane were permeable only to Na⁺ ions, these would enter the neuron until the resting potential settled at about +62 mV. If the plasma membrane were equally permeable to both K⁺ and Na⁺ ions, then the value of the membrane potential would be approximately equal to the difference of the two conducted potentials (about -18 mV). In reality, however, the neuron membrane is about 40 times more permeable to K⁺ ions than to Na⁺ ions, and therefore the resulting membrane potential of the neuron reaches a value of about -65 mV. This is due to the fact that the neuron membrane is highly permeable to K⁺ ions under resting conditions, the permeability to Na⁺ ions being significantly lower. The values of the resting membrane potential can be determined using the so-called Goldmann equation.

$$V_m = 61{,}5 \cdot \log \frac{P_{K^+}[K^+]_e + P_{Na^+}[Na^+]_e + P_{Cl^-}[Cl^-]_e}{P_{K^+}[K^+]_i + P_{Na^+}[Na^+]_i + P_{Cl^-}[Cl^-]_i}$$

This equation takes into account the relative permeability of the plasma membrane for several ions.

4.2 Excitability of neurons

Excitability is the property that allows a neuron to respond to a stimulus and transmit signals in electrical form. The transmission of signals within and between neurons is provided both electrically and chemically. The electrical signal, also referred to as the graded potential (receptor or generator, synaptic potential) and the action potential, are both the result of time-limited changes in the flow of current into and out of the neuron. These changes represent deviations from normal resting potential values. Ion channels in the plasma membrane regulate the flow of current in and out of the neuron. These channels exhibit three characteristics:

- are permeable to ions, and these ions can pass through them at high rates, up to 100×10^6 ions per second;
- are selectively permeable to certain ions;
- selectively open and close in response to specific electrical, chemical or mechanical stimuli.

Each neuron has more than 20 different types of ion channels, each of which can be found in thousands of copies in a given neuron. The passage of ions through ion channels is a passive process that requires no energy. The direction of passage of the ions is determined by the electrochemical forces acting across the plasma membrane.

One of the basic functions of ion channels in neurons is to mediate fast signaling. The channels, referred to as gated channels, contain a molecular closure, or gate, that opens rapidly and thus allows the passage of ions. Gating is the process by which a channel opens or closes as a result of the action of a particular stimulus. Most gated channels are closed under resting conditions.

Ligand-regulated channels open upon binding of a neurotransmitter molecule (or other chemical); voltage-regulated channels open and close in response to changes in membrane potential; modality-regulated channels are activated by specific stimuli (e.g., touch, pressure, stretch).

The energy required to open the gated channel comes from:
- from the binding of a neurotransmitter to a receptor protein that is part of ligand-regulated channels;
- from changes in the polarity of the plasma membrane in voltage-gated channels;
- from mechanical forces transmitted through interactions with the cytoskeleton at modality-controlled channels.

Two basic plasma membrane reactions are distinguished:
- hyperpolarisation, when the inner surface of the membrane becomes even more negative compared to the outer surface (e.g., potential change from -70 mV to -80 mV);
- depolarization, when the inner surface of the membrane becomes less negative compared to the outer surface, or a polarity reversal may occur when the inner membrane becomes positive relative to the outer membrane; this is referred to as depolarization as the membrane potential becomes less negative compared to the resting potential (e.g., from -70 mV to 0 to +40 mV).

5

Graded potential and action potential

Neurons are cells specialized in the production of electrical signals that are used to encode and transmit information. These signals are manifested by changes in resting membrane potential.

5.1 Graded potential

Voltage changes that are confined to the region where the stimulus is applied to the neuron (or in close proximity to this region) are referred to as graded potentials. These voltage changes can give rise to action potentials (nerve impulses) that transmit signals along axons over long distances. Two types of graded potentials are distinguished:

- generator potential, which is induced by the action of a sensory or sensory stimulus from the external or internal environment of the organism (sensory stimuli include pressure, tension, vibration, heat, cold, chemical substances; sensory stimuli act on the sensory organs - sight, smell, taste, hearing, balance);
- a synaptic potential that arises as part of the propagation of signals from one neuron to another neuron at the synapse, specifically at the postsynaptic membrane.

Both generator and synaptic potentials can give rise to an action potential, which in turn induces a synaptic potential on the next neuron it innervates. A synaptic potential evoked at a neuroeffector junction (e.g., neuromuscular disc, neuroglandular synapse) causes a response, which may be contraction of a muscle or release of substances by secretion from a glandular cell.

The generator and synaptic potentials differ from action potentials in that they encode some specific information. In addition, the graded potential encodes information in the analogue mode, i.e. it uses amplitude modulation (AM system), whereas the action potential encodes information in the digital mode and uses frequency modulation for encoding and transmission (FM system). The essence of the encoding of information in the generation of a graded potential is the fact that mild stimuli only induce a small potential (small voltage changes), whereas strong stimuli induce a large potential (large voltage changes). In both the central nervous system and autonomic ganglia, a mild depolarization (small voltage change), referred to as the excitatory postsynaptic potential (EPSP), occurs at the postsynaptic membrane of the excitatory synapse; a mild hyperpolarization, referred to as the inhibitory postsynaptic potential (IPSP), occurs at the postsynaptic membrane of the inhibitory synapse.

The basic characteristics of generator and synaptic potentials include:

- graded response - the magnitude of the response varies with the intensity of the stimulus; the more intense the stimulus, the greater the changes in membrane potential it produces;

- persistence of the response - the change in membrane potential can persist as long as the stimulus is applied;

- threshold for response - there is no set threshold; even the weakest stimuli can produce small changes in potential. Examples are small receptor potentials (rods or cones) or small synaptic potentials evoked by the action of a single photon or a few neurotransmitter molecules released from a single synaptic vesicle;

- response summation - potentials are summed when stimuli act in close succession or in close proximity to a given receptive segment of a neuron, with summation occurring both temporally and spatially;

- the response remains local - the potential propagates passively from the area of the stimulus (the point of origin); it is greatest at the point of origin, while its value gradually decreases with distance.

5.2 Action potential

In contrast to the generator and synaptic potentials, the action potential encodes information in a frequency-dependent manner. That is, a weak stimulus evokes only a few action potentials per given time unit, whereas a strong stimulus evokes action potentials at high frequency, but the signal amplitude is the same in both cases.

The basic characteristics of action potential include:

- all-or-nothing response - regardless of the stimulus intensity, the potential always has the same magnitude (range of changes around 100 mV);

- short-term response - the potentials have a constant duration (around 1.5 ms);

- threshold for response - activation leading to an action potential requires a significant change in membrane potential (more than 15 mV);

- size principle - smaller neurons need smaller EPSPs to reach the threshold for action potential generation than large neurons;

5. Graded potential and action potential

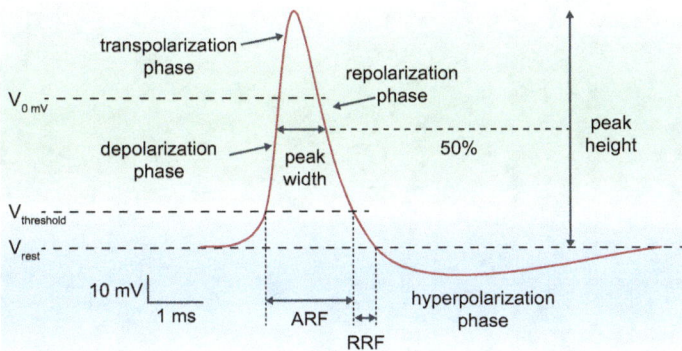

Figure 5.1 Schematic illustration of the basic characteristics of the action potential. When the value of the membrane potential in the region of the axon bump and the initial segment reaches a threshold level (a potential drop of approximately 15 mV), a nerve excitation occurs, the recording of which is referred to as an action potential. There is a rapid depolarization, or even an overshoot of the membrane potential to positive values (transpolarization). Subsequently, repolarization occurs, followed by a hyperpolarization phase. The absolute refractory phase (ARF) refers to the period when the neuronal membrane cannot be irritated, even by any intense suprathreshold stimulus. The ARF is followed by the relative refractory phase (RRF), when irritation can be induced, but only by application of an intense stimulus. RRF, threshold potential; V_{rest}, resting potential (modified according to Porth, 2004; Bean, 2007).

- refractory period - each action potential is followed by a period (about 1.5 ms) when the neuron is in a non-reactive phase; during this period no further action potentials are possible, regardless of the intensity of the applied stimulus;
- propagation of the response - the action potential involves a short-duration reverse current that is confined to a small area and that propagates in the form of a wave of depolarization along the axon; the action potential at the beginning of the axon (the site of origin) has the same amplitude as the action potential at the end of the axon; therefore, coding based on frequency changes (number of action potentials per unit time) is used as a neuronal code to transmit information; in addition, information is also coded by the pattern (sequence and spacing) of action potentials.

Part III. Signaling-related components of the neuron

A typical neuron is a cell that consists of a receptive segment, an initiating segment, a conducting segment, a transmission segment, and a trophic segment. Each of these segments show functional specialization (Fig. III.1).

The receptive segment is the area of the neuron that transforms stimuli or receives and integrates signals from many presynaptic neurons. This segment is specialized for the perception of stimuli (input), with the consequence of the action of the stimuli being the generation of a local potential. Each of the local potentials arising at synapses is the result of a transient change in the membrane potential in the immediate vicinity of the synapse at the receptive segment. The plasma membrane can respond by either depolarization or hyperpolarization, which is caused by a local change in permeability to certain ions (e.g., Na^+, K^+, and Cl^-). In those neurons where the dendrites and cell body form a receptive segment, the local potential is referred to as the synaptic (postsynaptic) potential or chemical potential. The channels involved in the generation of this potential are chemically (neurotransmitter) regulated (gated). In sensory neurons of peripheral nerves, the receptive segment is formed by a sensory receptor (e.g., a receptor for touch). This segment contains specific modality-regulated (gated) Na^+ and K^+ channels. In these neurons, local potentials are referred to as receptor or generator potentials, respectively.

The initiating segment is formed by a trigger region located between the receptive region and the conductive region. It is the region where the summation of the effects on the receptive region occurs and where the integrated potential is generated, which is capable of triggering the generation of an action potential in the conducting segment. The conducting segment is specialized for the transmission of nerve signals from the receptive segment to the transmitting segment. The conducting segment conducts all-or-nothing signals, i.e. action potentials (nerve impulses). This segment contains voltage-gated Na^+ and K^+ channels.

The transmission segment contains the presynaptic membrane and synaptic vesicles. The action potential transmitted by the conduction segment causes the release of neurotransmitter molecules through voltage-gated channels, which in turn affect the receptor segment of the next neuron or effector cell.

The trophic segment represents the body of the neuron, which is the metabolic center essential for maintaining neuronal viability. In most neurons, the trophic segment is located in the receptive segment. In sensory neurons of peripheral nerve, the cell body of the neuron is part of the conducting segment.

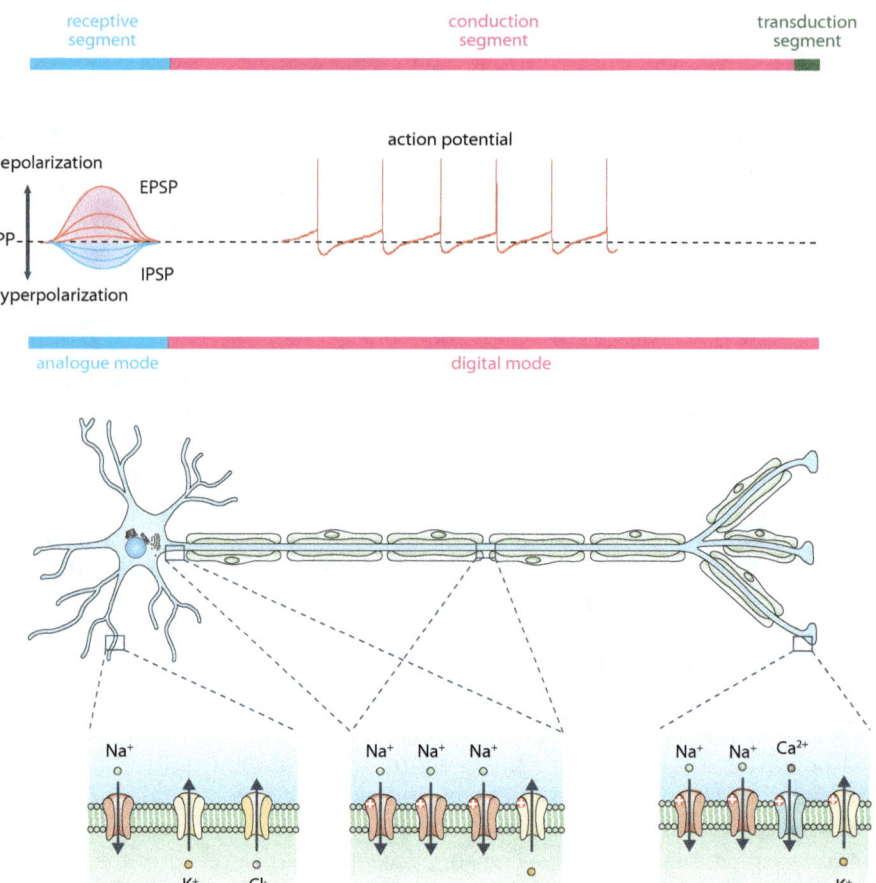

Figure III. 1 Schematic illustration of the structural and functional components (segments) of a representative neuron. The dendrites and body of the neuron represent the receptive segment that receives stimuli. The receptive segment is acted upon by stimuli that can induce changes in the membrane resting potential (PP) in terms of excitatory postsynaptic potential (EPSP) or inhibitory postsynaptic potential (IPSP). These potential changes are due to changes in membrane permeability mainly for Na^+, K^+ and Cl^- ions. The potential changes are summed, thus they are processed in the form of an analogue mode. If the changes in membrane polarity reach a threshold level, nerve excitations occur in the region of the axon initial segment. These are propagated through the conducting segment in digital mode. The digital mode is characterised by the fact that a subthreshold stimulus does not give rise to a nerve excitation, whereas a suprathreshold stimulus does. The amplitude of the action potential is constant and does not depend on the intensity of the suprathreshold stimulus. The conducting segment encodes the transmitted information in the frequency of the action potentials. The conducting segment, formed by the nerve ending, ensures the transmission of signals to the next neuron or effector cell. The membrane of individual neuron segments differs in the representation of ion channels, which determines the functional specialization of these segments (modified according to Noback et al., 2005).

6

Receptor segment and receptor potential

In most neurons, the receptive segment consists of dendrites and the cell body. In sensory neurons of peripheral nerve, the receptor segment is formed by that segment of the peripheral nerve ending located distal to the first node of Ranvier.

6.1 Dendrites and the cell body as a functional unit

The plasma membrane of the functional unit formed by the dendrites and the body of the neuron is the postsynaptic membrane, which is also referred to as the receptor membrane, since the permeability of the membrane is influenced by channels controlled by neurotransmitters that are released from the presynaptic nerve ending. Neurotransmitter-operated channels are permeable to ion pairs, either Na^+ and K^+ ions or K^+ and Cl^- ions. When these ion channels are activated, a reaction known as a receptor or synaptic potential is generated at the membrane, representing a graded response. Each graded reaction propagates as a potential along the plasma membrane over a small distance, persists for only 1 to 2 ms, and is not capable of generating an action potential on its own. However, if the stimuli act repeatedly over a short period of time, there is a summation of their effects as they reinforce or facilitate the graded response. There are no voltage-gated Na^+ and K^+ channels in the cell membrane in the region of dendrites and the cell body and therefore no action potential can arise there. Therefore, the action potential in most neurons arises in the region of the initiating segment, as this is the region of the cell membrane where a high concentration of voltage-gated Na^+ and K^+ channels are found.

Excitation of the receptor membrane results from a response to a neurotransmitter that partially depolarizes the postsynaptic membrane. This response is graded and is referred to as the excitatory postsynaptic potential (EPSP). The EPSP results from a change in the permeability of the postsynaptic membrane to Na^+ and K^+ ions, with Na^+ ions entering the neuron and K^+ ions leaving the neuron. A single EPSP is unable to reduce the membrane potential sufficiently to give rise to an action potential. In the case of multiple EPSPs arising simultaneously or in rapid succession, through facilitation, the membrane potential is lowered enough until an action potential arises in the initiating segment. The neurotransmitters that elicit EPSPs cause openings of both Na^+, and K^+ ion channels. The main excitatory neurotransmitters are glutamate and aspartate. Postsynaptic receptors binding these neurotransmitters are associated with ion channels for Na^+ and K^+. Thus, the entry of Na^+ ions into the neuron and the exit of K^+ ions from the neuron cause depolarization of the postsynaptic membrane and thus the formation of EPSP.

While the EPSP makes the neuron more likely to generate an action potential, the inhibitory postsynaptic potential (IPSP) does the opposite. Inhibition actually represents a hyperpolarization of the postsynaptic membrane in response to a neurotransmitter, where the voltage changes from, for example, -70 mV to -80 mV. The inhibitory response is the result of Cl^- ions entering the neuron and K^+ ions exiting the neuron through the postsynaptic membrane ion channels that are controlled by the neurotransmitter. The main inhibitory neurotransmitters are GABA and glycine. The postsynaptic receptors binding these neurotransmitters are associated with ion channels for Cl^-. Thus, the resulting entry of Cl^- ions into the neuron causes hyperpolarization of the postsynaptic membrane and thus the formation of IPSPs.

A large number of ion channels controlled by excitatory or inhibitory neurotransmitters can be found in the postsynaptic membrane of a neuron. Both types of channels are capable of altering the membrane permeability of the receptor segment of the neuron. The integration of these changes is a property of the dendrite and the body of the neuron. In case the excitatory activity reaches the necessary threshold, an action potential is generated.

In general, excitatory synapses eliciting EPSP are found in greater abundance on dendrites, whereas inhibitory synapses are more commonly formed on the body of the neuron. The aforementioned differential spatial representation of excitatory and inhibitory synapses is of functional significance. EPSPs can aggregate on dendrites and, to a lesser extent, on the cell body, thereby inducing excitation of the neuron. In contrast, IPSPs, by arising closer to the initiating segment, may thus effectively regulate the extent of excitatory action on the axon initiating segment and thus the generation of action potentials.

6.2 Receptive segment of peripheral sensory and sensory neurons

Sensory neurons, which transmit signals from the body's external and internal environment via peripheral nerves to the central nervous system, have a specific structural arrangement The peripheral sensory endings of these fibers, many of which make contacts with specialized cells (e.g. the Corti spiral organ in the inner ear or neuromuscular spindles in muscles), have a short receptive segment. The plasma membrane of this segment contains Na^+ and K^+ channels controlled by specific modalities. The action of these modalities gives rise to receptor or generator potentials. Pressure acting on touch receptors or stretching of muscle spindles acting on sensory endings cause the opening of the above ion channels. When the generator potential reaches the region of the first Ranvier node (analogous to the initiating segment in other neurons), an action potential is generated.

7

Initial and conductive segment

While the initiating segment is where action potentials are formed, the conducting segment (axon) is specialized for the transmission of action potentials, often over longer distances.

7.1 Initial segment and integrated potential

The axon initiation segment in most neurons, or the region of the first Ranvier node of peripheral sensory neurons, represents a specialized segment where the action potential arises. That segment of the neuron's membrane represents the integrating region where the (algebraic) summation of EPSPs and IPSPs arising on the receptive (synaptic) segment occurs. The initiating segment is also referred to as the trigger zone or the zone of action potential (impulse) generation, because it is in this region that action potentials are generated and subsequently conducted through the axon. Action potentials arise in the initiating segment because this section of the membrane has a low threshold (approximately -45 mV) for depolarization to occur. If the integrated potential reaches the threshold, a discharge or action potential will occur.

Each receptor converts the energy of the applied stimulus (mechanical, electromagnetic, thermal, chemical) into electrochemical changes in the neuron and thus transforms the diverse stimuli into a single, common "language" (action potential) that is the same for all sensory modalities. This signal is subsequently transmitted through the conducting segment.

7.2 Conducting segment and action potential

The conduction segment is the part of the neuron that is specialized for the transmission of action potentials (nerve impulses), i.e. fast propagating waves of electrical excitation that propagate across the axon membrane without changing amplitude (all-or-nothing digital mode). Based on the shape of the curve showing

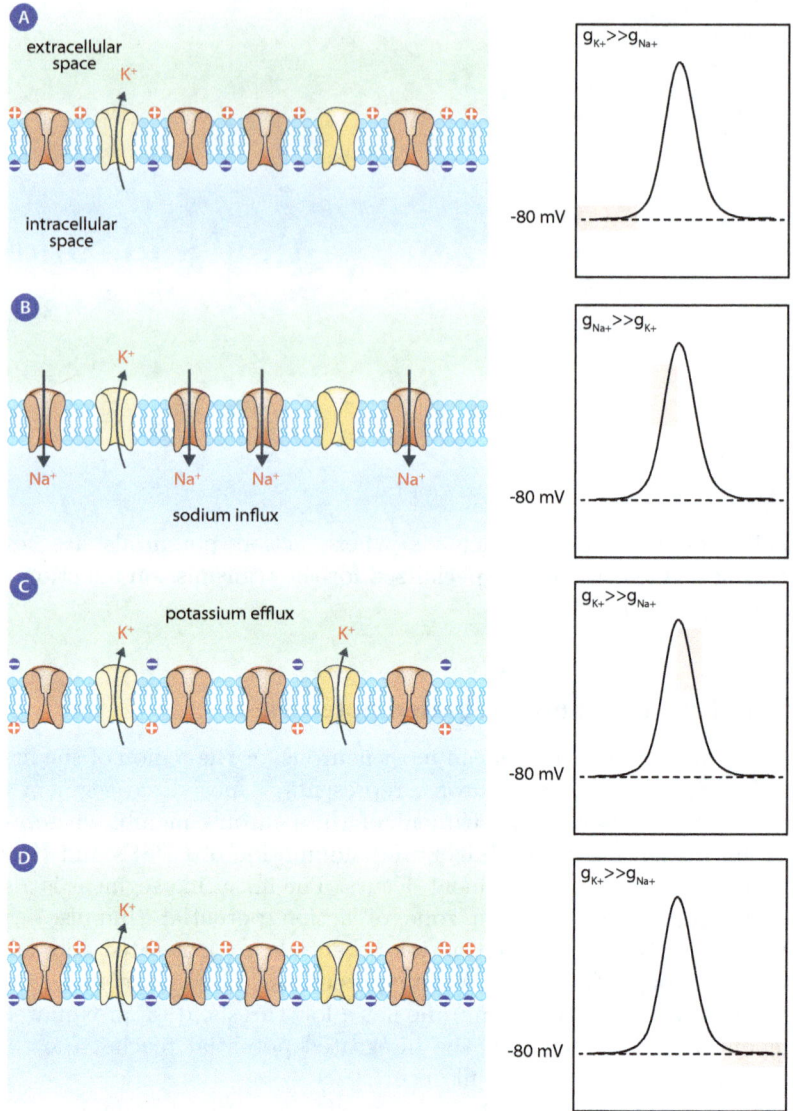

Figure 7.1 Schematic illustration of the changes in axon membrane permeability that underlie action potential propagation. During rest, the axon membrane is permeable to K$^+$ ions (A). During propagation of the nerve impulse along the axon, voltage-gated channels for Na$^+$ ions open due to changes in membrane polarity (B). The passage of these ions into the neuron causes depolarization. With a certain latency, voltage-gated channels for K$^+$ ions open, which, together with the gradual closure of channels for Na$^+$ ions, causes the membrane polarity to return to resting values (C-D). g_K - membrane conductance for K$^+$ ions; g_{Na} - membrane conductance for Na$^+$ ions (modified according to Govindarajan et al., 2006; Bear et al., 2015).

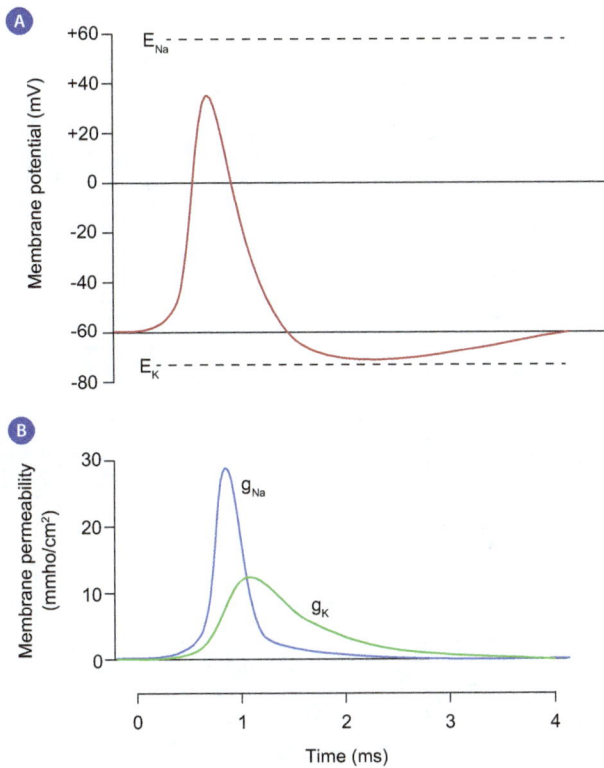

Figure 7.2 Schematic illustration of the changes in membrane potential and axon membrane permeability that give rise to the action potential. The generation and propagation of nerve excitations result from precisely timed changes in the permeability of voltage-gated channels for Na$^+$ and K$^+$ ions. EK - equilibrium potential for K$^+$ ions; ENa - equilibrium potential for Na$^+$ ions; g_K - membrane conductance for K$^+$ ions; g_{Na} - membrane conductance for Na$^+$ ions (modified according to Javorka et al., 2009).

the changes in membrane potential, action potentials are also referred to as spike potentials. The all-or-nothing mode means that the pulse is either present and then propagates without a change in amplitude, or it is not present. The occurrence of an action potential results from the action of the integrating potential of the initiating segment, which in turn activates the voltage-gated ion channels of the conducting segment of the neuron. The result is a change in the permeability of the cell membrane to Na$^+$ and K$^+$ ions. If the applied stimulus causes the resting potential of the axon to fall below a critical level, usually 10 to 15 mV less than the resting potential value, a massive change occurs that is caused by the opening of voltage-gated ion channels of the conducting segment of the neuron. This results in the generation of an action potential, which is a manifestation of graded depolarization. Depolarization results from changes in membrane permeability caused by the opening of voltage-gated ion channels Na$^+$ and K$^+$. Within a few milliseconds there is a reversal of polarity from a resting potential of -60 to -70 mV to +30 mV, when a negative charge predominates on the extracellular side of the

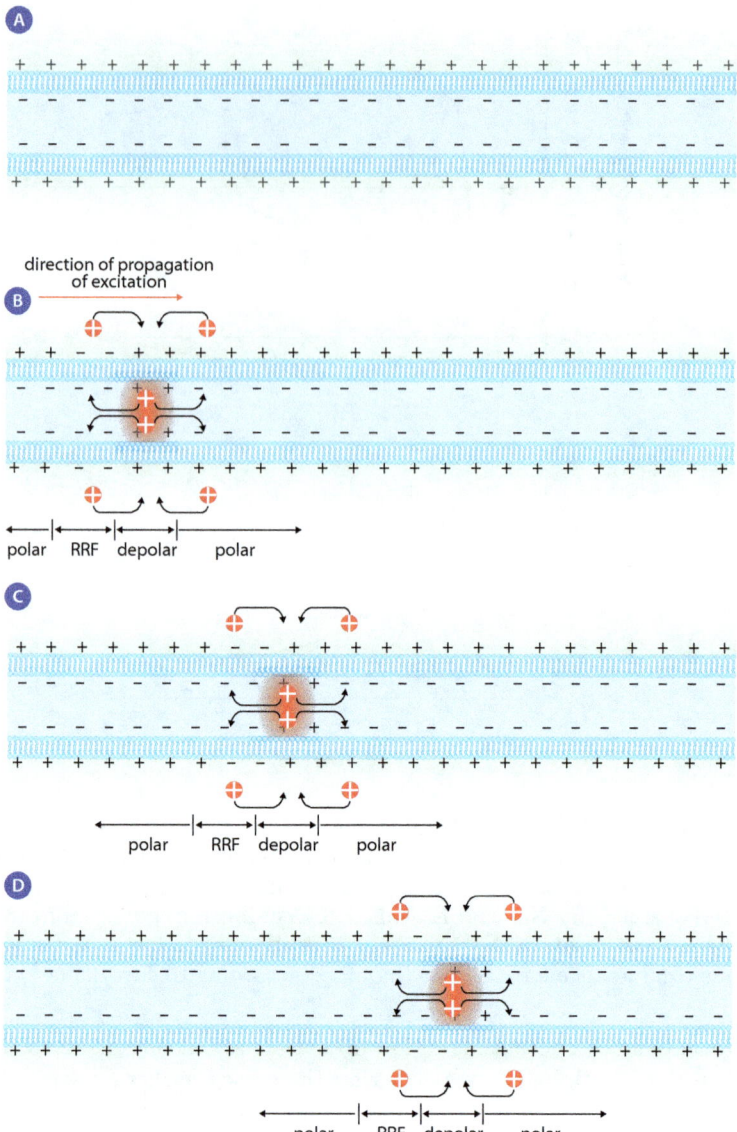

Figure 7.3 Schematic illustration of the propagation of nerve excitation in an unmyelinated axon. Under resting conditions, the plasma membrane of the axon is polarized (A). The nerve excitation propagates in the form of a depolarization wave (B-D). Back-propagation of the nerve excitation is prevented by the relative refractory phase (RRF) in which the previously depolarized membrane is located. Depolar, depolarized membrane; polar, polarized membrane (modified according to Javorka et al., 2009).

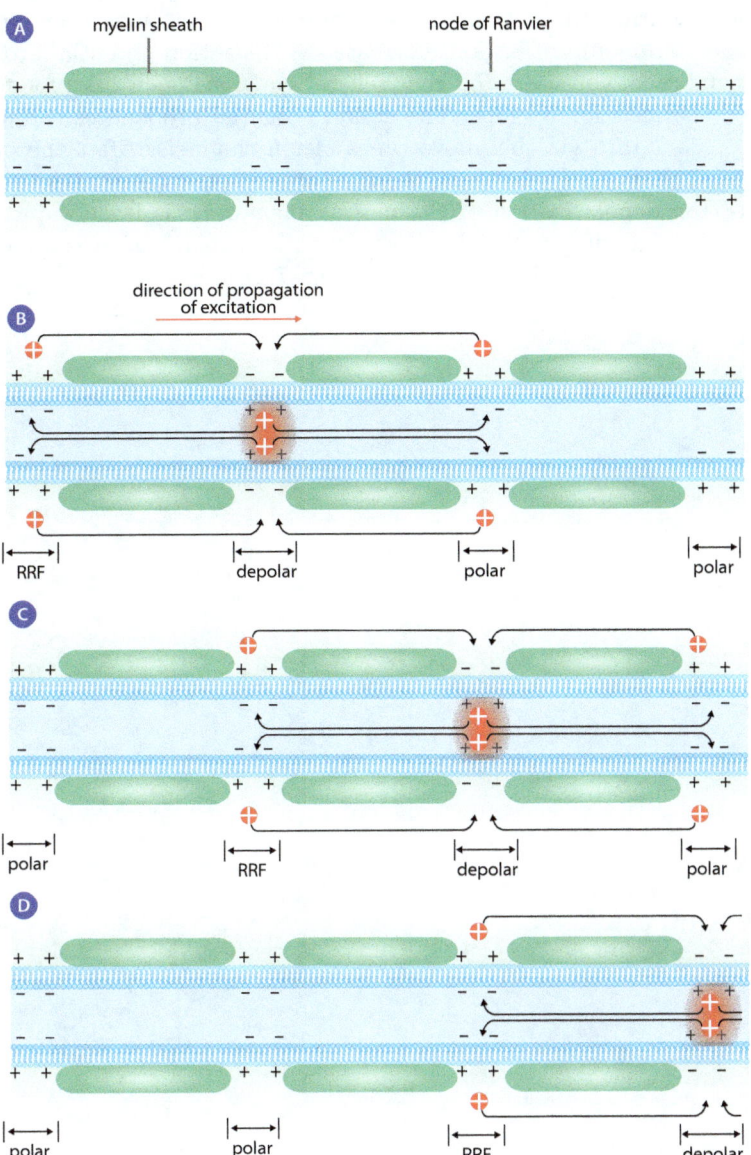

Figure 7.4 Schematic illustration of the propagation of nerve excitation in a myelinated axon. Under resting conditions, the plasma membrane of the axon is polarized (A). Nerve excitation propagates saltatory, in the form of depolarization jumps (B-D). Backward propagation of the nerve excitation is prevented by the relative refractory phase (RRF) in which the previously depolarized membrane is located. Depolar, depolarized membrane; polar, polarized membrane (modified according to Purves et al., 2008).

cell membrane. During the action potential transition, Na^+ ions accumulate in the axon while the amount of K^+ ions decrease. As the action potential progresses across the membrane, voltage-gated channels for Na^+ ions open first, followed by voltage-gated channels for K^+ ions. The action potential propagates through the axon at a constant rate via the above types of ion channels. After the opening of voltage-gated channels for K^+ ions, the membrane potential returns to resting values. Thus, the depolarization of the plasma membrane is largely due to the change in its permeability to Na^+ ions, whereas the repolarization is largely due to the change in its permeability to K^+ ions (Fig. 7.1).

8

Transduction (synaptic or effector) segment

A transmission or synaptic segment is the part(s) of a neuron through which it influences the activity of other neurons or effector cells (e.g., myocytes, gland cells). Structurally, it is formed by the presynaptic portion of the synapse, which includes the presynaptic membrane and vesicles containing neurotransmitters or their precursors.

Action potential transmission to the transduction segment region activates voltage-gated channels for Ca^{2+} ions located on the presynaptic membrane, resulting in the movement of Ca^{2+} ions into the neuron. The rise in the concentration of Ca^{2+} ions in the transfer segment represents the key final event underlying neurotransmitter release into the synaptic cleft. Voltage-gated channels for Ca^{2+} ions regulate the basic, secretory function of the neuron.

The synapse (of the chemical type) functions as a one-way valve that allows the action potential of the activated neuron to influence, through the release of neurotransmitters and their diffusion across the synaptic cleft, the receptive segment of the innervated neuron (or effector cell). An exception is the axo-axonal synapse, where two transmission segments are in contact and which is involved in processes associated with presynaptic inhibition or presynaptic excitation.

A delay is present between the arrival of the action potential at the transduction segment of the neuron and the release of neurotransmitters, which is caused by the time required for Ca^{2+} ions to pass into the presynaptic termination and the subsequent molecular events that lead to the actual release of the synaptic vesicle contents into the synaptic cleft.

8.1 Neuromuscular junction (disc)

The synapse at the motor plate formed by the axon termination and the plasma membrane of the skeletal muscle fiber (sarcolemma) is an example of the regulation of effector cell activity by neurons. Transmission of the action potential to the presynaptic ending causes the release of the neurotransmitter acetylcholine, which binds to nicotinic-type cholinergic receptors present in the sarcolemma. This leads to the generation of a plate potential that causes depolarization of the sarcolemma in close proximity to the neuromuscular disc. The depolarization causes the opening of voltage-gated channels for Na^+ and K^+ ions in the sarcolemma and the generation of an action potential. The action potential is rapidly conducted along the surface of the myocyte as well as to the inner parts through the membranes of numerous transverse tubules. The action potential stimulates the release of Ca^{2+} ions from the sarcoplasmic reticulum, which initiate processes associated with contraction of the myocyte as a whole. Movement of Ca^{2+} ions into the sarcoplasmic reticulum results in relaxation of the myocyte.

Part IV. Synaptic transmission and neurotransmission

The transmission of signals between neurons and between neurons and effector cells is mediated by neurotransmitters and neuromodulators that are released from axon endings (and possibly also from dendrites). Morphologically and functionally, there are two basic types of signal transduction, each of which exhibits several variations (Fig. IV.1).

Wiring transmission is a signal transmission mechanism based on relatively close contact between the structures of two neurons, involving:

- chemical synapse - the signal transmission takes place from one axon ending of a neuron to another neuron, while the signal transmission is mostly unidirectional;

- electrical synapse - signal transmission takes place between two neurons, and the transmission can take place in both directions;

- juxtaposition of membranes - electrical potentials allow mutual modulation of excitability of membranes of neurons that are in close proximity.

Volume transmission is a mechanism for the transmission of signals via molecules released from axon terminals into the surroundings of the neuron, outside the synaptic cleft, whereby a single neuron can influence the activity of a larger number of surrounding neurons. This mechanism includes:

- extrasynaptic release - the released neurotransmitter diffuses around the synapse and acts on receptors in its vicinity;

- the released neurotransmitter passes into the circulation - for example, hypothalamic liberins and statins;

- the released neurotransmitters pass into the cerebral ventricles, in which cerebrospinal fluid circulates, allowing the neurotransmitter to act in a remote area of the nervous system;

- en passant synapse, when the classical synaptic conformation is not formed - the released neurotransmitter freely diffuses into the surroundings and thus influences the activity of a larger number of neurons;

- circulating substances can modify the activity of neurons - predominantly in the circumventricular organs of the brain.

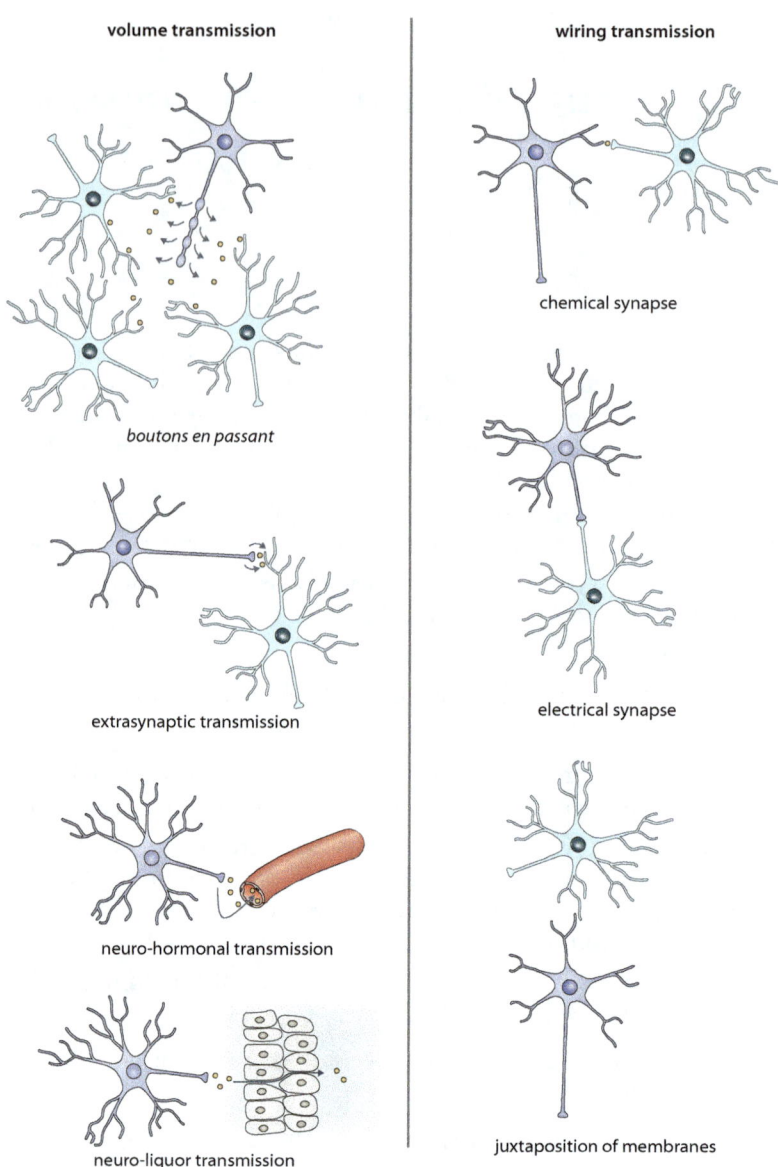

Figure IV.1 Schematic illustration of the different types of communication in the nervous system. The cross-linked type of transmission is conditioned by the relatively close proximity of the neuronal processes, with signal transmission taking place from one process to the other process. In volume signal transmission, the neurons that communicate with each other are relatively distant, with signal transmission often taking place from one nerve ending to a large number of other neurons (modified according to Agnati et al., 1995; Sykova, 2004).

9

Chemical synapses

The vast majority of synaptic connections in the nervous system are of the chemical synapse type. The processes involved in transmission at a chemical synapse can be divided into four steps:
- neurotransmitter synthesis;
- neurotransmitter storage and release;
- interaction of the transmitter with the receptors;
- removal and reuse of neurotransmitter and synaptic vesicles (Fig. 9.1).

Similarly, the above processes also take place in synapses formed between the neuron and the effector cell (e.g. neuromuscular disc).

Neurons use two basic types of molecules, small molecule neurotransmitters and neuropeptides, to transmit signals at chemical synapses.

9.1 Synthesis of neurotransmitters

Synthesis of small-molecule neurotransmitters can take place in all parts of neurons, but it occurs predominantly in the presynaptic ending where the necessary enzymes are located, and the synthesized neurotransmitters are subsequently placed in synaptic vesicles. In contrast to small molecule neurotransmitters, neuropeptides are synthesized in the body of the neuron, where the necessary proteosynthetic apparatus is located.

9.2 Storage and release of neurotransmitters

The synthesized neurotransmitters are immediately placed into vesicles, which are anchored via the cytoskeleton and located in the "reserve" zone of the nerve ending filled with vesicles. If a neurotransmitter molecule is released into the cytoplasm, degradation can occur. Thus, vesicles represent a reservoir of neurotransmitters, protecting them from the action of cytoplasmic enzymes. Small-molecule neurotransmitters are stored in small, transparent vesicles about

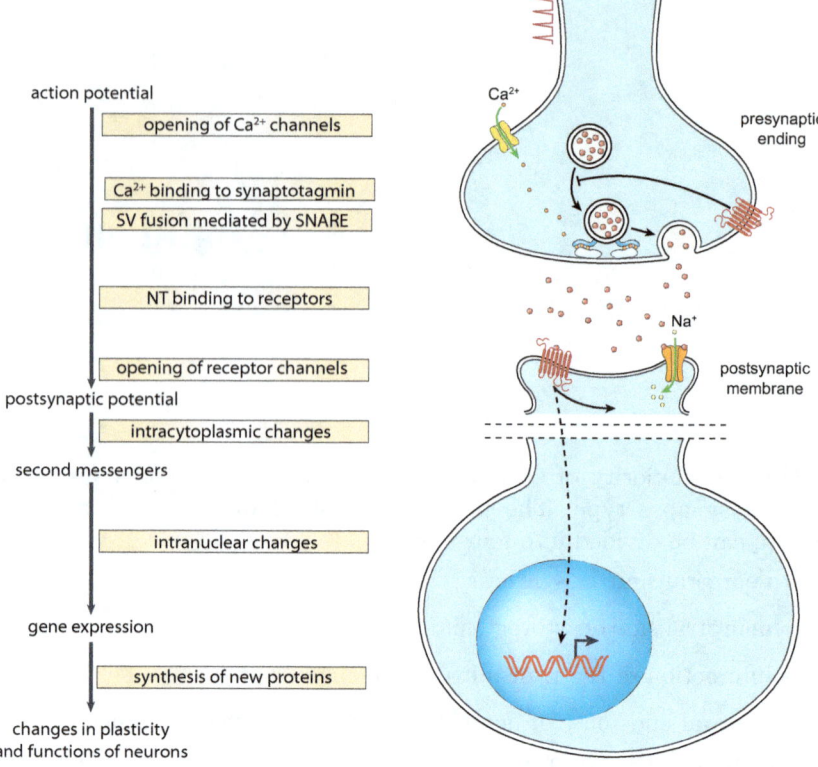

Figure 9.1 Schematic illustration of the basic processes that take place at a chemical synapse from which small-molecule neurotransmitters are released. Enzymes in the nerve ending synthesize the neurotransmitter, which is stored in secretory vesicles. After depolarization of the presynaptic area by the action potential, there is a rise in the intracellular concentration of Ca^{2+} ions. The increased concentration of calcium in the presynaptic region triggers a cascade of events resulting in fusion of the vesicles containing the neurotransmitter with the presynaptic membrane of the neuron, thereby releasing the neurotransmitter into the synaptic cleft. The neurotransmitter acts on postsynaptically localized ionotropic or metabotropic receptors, thereby inducing changes in the postsynaptic membrane (depolarization or hyperpolarization), but it can also affect intracellular events that may result, for example, in a change in gene expression of the neuron. At the same time, the neurotransmitter may also act on presynaptically localized autoreceptors. The action of a neurotransmitter is terminated by its degradation in the synaptic cleft (e.g., acetylcholine) or by its reuptake into the presynaptic nerve ending (e.g., monoamines) or by glia cells (e.g., glutamate). The neurotransmitter recaptured into the nerve ending is either metabolized or can be released back into the synaptic cleft after storage in secretory vesicles. NT, neurotransmitter; SV, synaptic vesicles; SNAREs, proteins responsible for the fusion of vesicle membranes (containing neurotransmitters) with the plasma membrane of the presynaptic nerve ending (modified according to Ribrault et al., 2011; Popoli et al., 2012; Purves et al., 2017).

50 nm in diameter. From the reserve region, the vesicles are translocated to the active zone of the presynaptic terminus, where they are anchored with a complex of "fusion pore" proteins. The entry of Ca^{2+} ions into the nerve ending causes the vesicles to fuse with the presynaptic membrane and release the neurotransmitter into the synaptic cleft. Ca^{2+} ions also mobilize vesicles anchored to components of the cytoskeleton and allow their anchoring and binding to the "fusion pore" protein complex.

Unlike small-molecule neurotransmitters, neuropeptide precursors are synthesized and stored in secretory granules and synaptic vesicles in the body of the neuron, where the necessary synthetic apparatus (e.g., cell nucleus, ribosomes, endoplasmic reticulum, and Golgi apparatus) is located. They are subsequently transported by rapid axonal transport via neurotubules to the axon terminal. Neuropeptides are stored in large (electron-dense) vesicles about 120 nm in diameter.

Small-molecule neurotransmitters and neuropeptides can co-occur in a single presynaptic ending. The joint release of multiple neurotransmitters from the presynaptic ending and the presence of corresponding receptors on the postsynaptic membrane provide the basis for the transmission of different signals at a single synapse.

9.3 Binding of neurotransmitters to receptors

The released neurotransmitter diffuses across the synaptic cleft and binds to specific receptors located on the postsynaptic membrane, initiating a cascade of subsequent changes. Based on the effects, molecules released from the presynaptic ending are divided into neurotransmitters and neuromodulators.

Neurotransmitters are molecules that directly affect ion channels on the postsynaptic membrane because they bind to receptors of which the ion channels are an integral part (called ionotropic receptors) (Fig. 9.2). The binding of a neurotransmitter to an ionotropic receptor, first of all, induces a change in the permeability of the ion channel that is part of the receptor. This results in a relatively rapid change in the polarity of the postsynaptic membrane. Neurotransmitters that bind to ionotropic receptors include acetylcholine, glutamate, aspartate, GABA, and glycine. By binding to these receptors, they rapidly induce the formation of EPSP or IPSP. These local potentials arise in fractions of milliseconds after neurotransmitter release and rarely persist longer than 100 ms. While glutamate and aspartate, as excitatory neurotransmitters, elicit EPSP, GABA and glycine, inhibitory neurotransmitters, elicit the induction of IPSP. Acetylcholine can act as both an excitatory and an inhibitory neurotransmitter, depending on the type of receptor to which it binds.

Neuromodulators are those molecules that modify or modulate nerve activity rather than directly leading to the generation of nerve impulses (action potentials). Binding of a neuromodulator to a metabotropic receptor induces a cascade of changes via G proteins and subsequently second messengers, which also results in a change in ion channel permeability (Fig. 9.3). Their effects are delayed in onset but can persist for several seconds to hours or even longer. Neuromodulators include the monoamines dopamine, norepinephrine, epinephrine, serotonin and

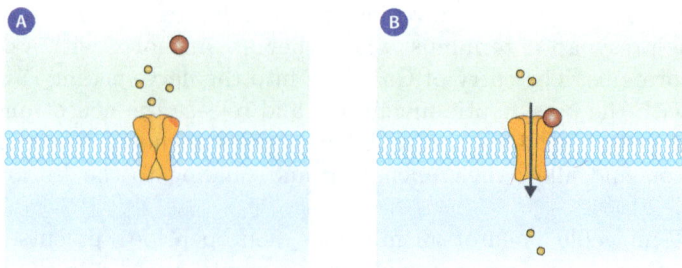

Figure 9.2 Schematic illustration of ionotropic receptor activation. Occupancy of the ionotropic receptor leads to a conformational change resulting in the change plasma membrane permeability for ions (modified according to Mombaerts, 2004; Purves et al., 2008).

histamine as well as neuropeptides. In the following, the uniform designation neurotransmitters is also used for chemicals in the neuromodulator group.

Activation of ionotropic and metabotropic receptors induces other events (from activation of protein kinases to changes in gene expression) in addition to changes in ion channel permeability and subsequent changes in the polarity of neuronal membranes. These are mostly events that take place with a certain latency and often persist for a longer period of time, compared to changes in membrane polarity. Examples are gaseous neurotransmitters, which can exert their effect by binding to the intracellularly localized enzyme guanylate cyclase.

This classification on neurotransmitters and neuromodulators is not absolute, however, as several neurotransmitters act on both ionotropic and metabotropic receptors (e.g., acetylcholine, glutamate). Acetylcholine released from preganglionic neurons in the autonomic ganglia or from motor neurons of the anterior horns of the spinal cord in the area of the neuromuscular disc, after binding to ionotropic (nicotinic) receptors, induces rapid excitation of postganglionic autonomic neurons or contraction of striated muscle. In the brain and in internal organs (e.g., heart), however, acetylcholine, by binding to metabotropic (muscarinic) receptors, can induce a slower and longer-lasting, modulatory change on postsynaptic neurons.

Neurosteroids act by binding to intracellular receptors and induce changes that take time to become apparent and may persist for prolonged periods of time. This may involve the formation of new proteins, e.g. receptors, ion channels. In contrast, binding to membrane receptors can induce relatively rapid changes in neuronal activity by affecting the activity of receptors for other neurotransmitters (e.g., $GABA_A$ receptors). Neurosteroids may act not only through binding to intracellular receptors, but also through binding to membrane receptors for other neurotransmitters. It is thought that the rapid effect of neurosteroids may be mediated by receptors coupled to G proteins.

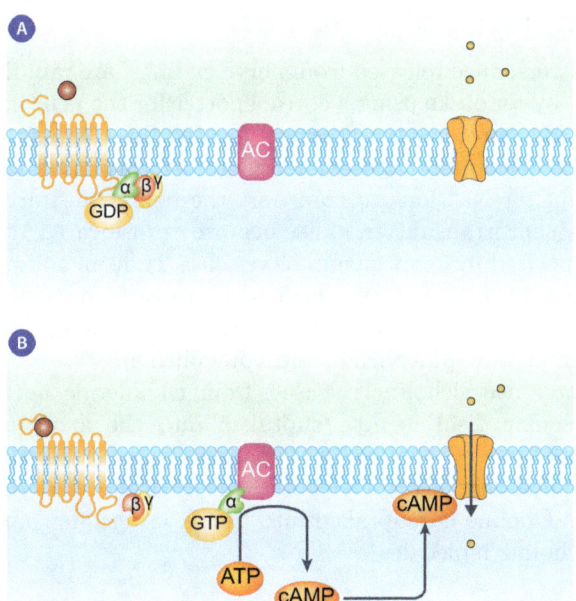

Figure 9.3 Schematic illustration of metabotropic receptor activation. Occupancy of the metabotropic receptor leads to activation of the G protein (composed of α and βγ subunits). G protein activation subsequently modifies intracellular processes via second messengers. These events can result not only in a change in neuronal excitability but also in gene expression. In the above case, the binding of the neurotransmitter with a metabotropic receptor leads to the activation of Gs protein, which induces the production of cAMP by the enzyme adenylate cyclase (AC). cAMP affects ion channel permeability (modified according to Mombaerts, 2004; Purves et al., 2008).

9.4 Removal and recycling of synaptic vesicles and neurotransmitters

9.4.1 Vesicle membranes

The release of the neurotransmitter into the synaptic cleft is the result of the fusion of vesicles (containing the neurotransmitter) with the presynaptic membrane. After neurotransmitter release via exocytosis, the vesicle membrane becomes part of the presynaptic membrane, being coated on the inner surface with a dense layer of clathrin protein. The coated membrane is subsequently released back into the presynaptic ending by the process of endocytosis. The clathrin layer is enzymatically removed from the vesicle surface within seconds. Most recycled membranes form transitional structures, referred to as cisternae, before being refilled with neurotransmitter molecules.

9.4.2 Neurotransmitter removal and reuptake

Most neurotransmitters, once released from nerve endings, are rapidly removed from the synaptic cleft by reuptake using a cotransporter for the neurotransmitter and Na^+ ions. This glycoprotein transporter, located in the axon terminal membrane or in the glia cell membrane, uses energy in the form of a transmembrane electrochemical gradient for Na^+ ions to transport the neurotransmitter back to the neuron. Once the neurotransmitter molecules are translocated to the axon terminals, they are deposited into new synaptic vesicles. Transmembrane transfer that is specific to the neurotransmitters ensures reuptake of neurotransmitters such as glutamate, aspartate, glycine, GABA, serotonin, histamine, and the catecholamines (dopamine, norepinephrine, and epinephrine).

The neurotransmitter acetylcholine released from cholinergic nerve endings (e.g. in the neuromuscular disc) is not reuptaken into the axon ending. On the postsynaptic membrane of cholinergic synapses is localized the enzyme acetylcholinesterase, which degrades acetylcholine released into the synaptic cleft to choline and acetate. Choline is reuptaken into the axon terminals and used to synthesize new acetylcholine molecules.

10

Neurotransmitters and neuromodulators

The nervous system uses a wide range of neurotransmitters and neuromodulators to transmit signals. There are currently between 50 and 100 known substances from different chemical groups that meet some or all of the criteria for classification as neurotransmitters or neuromodulators (Table 10.1). This diversity allows for the complexity of signal processing in the nervous system (Webster, 2001).

The classification of neurotransmitters into different groups on the basis of selected characteristics is often used, but it is rather didactic.
According to the nature of the response elicited on the postsynaptic neuron, neurotransmitters can be divided into three groups:
- excitatory (e.g., glutamate and aspartate),
- inhibitory (e.g., GABA and glycine),
- modulatory (acetylcholine, norepinephrine, epinephrine, dopamine, serotonin and histamine).

According to the size of the molecule, neurotransmitters can be divided into two large groups:
- neurotransmitters with "small" molecular weight (e.g., amino acids, monoamines) (Tab. 10.1),
- neurotransmitters with "large" molecular weight (neuropeptides) (Tab. 10.2).

10.1 Effects of neurotransmitters

Neurotransmitters can produce multiple effects:
- changes in the postsynaptic membrane:
  - depolarization of the postsynaptic membrane;
  - hyperpolarization of the postsynaptic membrane.

Chemical group	Example (abbreviation)
choline ester	acetylcholine (Ach)
monoamines	
catecholamines	dopamine norepinephrine epinephrine
indoles	serotonin (5-hydroxytryptamine, 5-HT)
imidazoles	histamine (Hist)
amino acids	
excitatory	glutamate (Glu) aspartate (Asp)†
inhibitory	γ-aminobutyric acid (GABA) glycine (Gly)
purines	adenosine (A) adenosine triphosphate (ATP)
steroids	pregnenolone (Preg) dehydroepiandrosterone (DHEA)
gaseous substances	nitric oxide (NO) carbon monoxide (CO) hydrogen sulfide (H2S)
eicosanoids	prostaglandins (PG)

Table 10.1 Overview of small molecule neurotransmitter or neuromodulator groups. Acetylcholine, monoamines, and amino acids are among the "classical" neurotransmitters that fulfill all the basic characteristics of neurotransmitters. Purines, steroids, gaseous substances and eicosanoids are neuromodulators with specific properties.

Depolarization or hyperpolarization of the postsynaptic membrane is one of the basic manifestations of the action of neurotransmitters. On the basis of this effect, neurotransmitters can therefore be divided into excitatory and inhibitory. However, some neurotransmitters act by predominantly modulating the excitability of the postsynaptic membrane. These are referred to as modulatory.

- changes in gene expression in the neuron. Neurotransmitters can induce phosphorylation of transcriptional proteins via second messengers. The phosphorylated transcription factors subsequently modify gene expression in the neuron. The modified gene expression results in the synthesis of new proteins (Fig. 10.1). This type of neurotransmitter action induces changes that persist for days to months. Such long-term changes are likely to be important for processes such as neuronal development and long-term memory formation. Neurotransmitters can induce local protein synthesis in specific dendritic spines. This is thought to be a mechanism involved in the long-term structural and functional changes of the synapse.
- trophic effects. An example is GABA, which during nervous system maturation affects proliferation, migration and differentiation of nervous system cells, synapse maturation and cell death.
- changes in the presynaptic membrane. Presynaptically localized receptors

for a neurotransmitter that is released from the same presynaptic nerve ending are referred to as presynaptic autoreceptors. Receptors localized on the presynaptic membrane but occupied by a neurotransmitter released from a different nerve ending are referred to as presynaptic heteroreceptors. Autoreceptors and heteroreceptors located on the presynaptic nerve ending modulate the release of neurotransmitters from that nerve ending. Occupation of these receptors by their agonists largely causes a decrease in neurotransmitter release. Activation of autoreceptors by the released neurotransmitter therefore acts as a negative feedback that inhibits further neurotransmitter release. Presynaptically localized heteroreceptors allow complex interactions between different neurotransmitter systems, resulting in precise regulation of neurotransmitter release in the nervous system.

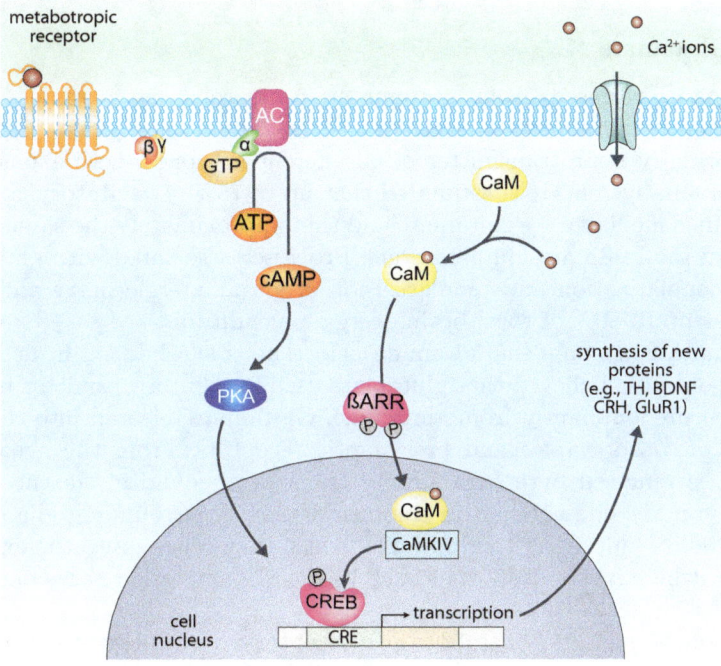

Figure 10.1 Schematic illustration of the influence of neurotransmitters on gene expression in a neuron. Activation of predominantly metabotropic receptors conditions a cascade of cytoplasmic changes. As a result, gene expression is activated and new proteins are produced, which may be enzymes of neurotransmitter biosynthesis, receptors for neurotransmitters as well as growth factors. In contrast to the action of excitatory and inhibitory neurotransmitters, which induce relatively short-lived changes in plasma membrane polarity, modulatory neurotransmitters, by affecting gene expression, induce changes that persist for many times longer. AC, adenylate cyclase; ATP, adenosine triphosphate; BDNF, brain-derived neurotrophic factor; CaM, calmodulin; CaMKIV, calmodulin-dependent kinase IV; cAMP, cyclic adenosine monophosphate; CREB, cAMP-responsive element; CRH, corticoliberin; GluR1, glutamate receptor subunit; GTP, guanosine diphosphate; PKA, protein kinase A; TH, tyrosine hydroxylase (modified according to Kandel et al., 2000; West et al., 2002; Carlezon et al., 2005).

10.2 Small molecule neurotransmitters

Among the first neurotransmitters to be identified are acetylcholine, biogenic amines, and some amino acids. Later, this group of small-molecule neurotransmitters grew to include purines, neurosteroids, cannabinoids, and other substances.

10.2.1 Excitatory amino acids

The excitatory amino acids glutamate and aspartate, by binding to metabotropic receptors, induce rapid changes in the electrical potential of the postsynaptic membrane. However, these neurotransmitters can also bind to metabotropic receptors.

10.2.1.1 Glutamate

Glutamate, released from glutamatergic neurons, is a major excitatory neurotransmitter in almost all areas of the central nervous system. Glutamate is also the primary neurotransmitter of all afferent neurons whose axons enter the central nervous system. It is estimated that up to 75% of excitatory transmission in the brain is mediated by glutamate and that approximately the same amount of synapses in the brain are glutamatergic. Processes associated with glutamatergic activity (depolarization and repolarization of glutamatergic nerve endings) may account for up to 80% of total brain energy expenditure.

Glutamate is a non-essential amino acid that is synthesized in neurons from its precursors. It is believed that glutamate used for neurotransmitter functions is synthesized predominantly from glutamine. Glutamate released into the synaptic cleft acts on postsynaptic and presynaptic receptors. From the synaptic cleft, glutamate is removed by a high-affinity transporter found in the membranes of presynaptic nerve endings and in the membranes of surrounding glia cells. Glial cells metabolize glutamate to glutamine, which they release into the extracellular fluid, from where it is transported back to the glutamatergic nerve endings (Fig. 10.2).

Both ionotropic and metabotropic receptors for glutamate are found in the central nervous system. Glutamate, after binding to ionotropic receptors, increases cation transfer, thereby participating in the excitation of postsynaptic neurons. The ionotropic receptors for glutamate include AMPA (the agonist is γ-amino-3-hydroxy-5-methyl-4-isoxazolepropionic acid), NMDA (the agonist is N-methyl d-aspartate), and kainate receptors. The AMPA and kainate receptors include "simple" cation channels that allow the passage of Na^+ ions intracellularly and K^+ ions extracellularly. The NMDA receptor exhibits several specificities. It is a receptor that also includes a cation channel, but which allows the transfer of relatively large amounts of Ca^{2+} ions into neuron. NMDA receptor function is facilitated by glycine binding, and it is this process that appears to be very important for the normal response of this ionotropic receptor to glutamate. Additionally, at resting membrane potential, the NMDA receptor ion channel is blocked by Mg^{2+} ions. Unblocking of the NMDA receptor (removal of Mg^{2+} ions) occurs only when the neuronal membrane is depolarized. Ionotropic glutamate

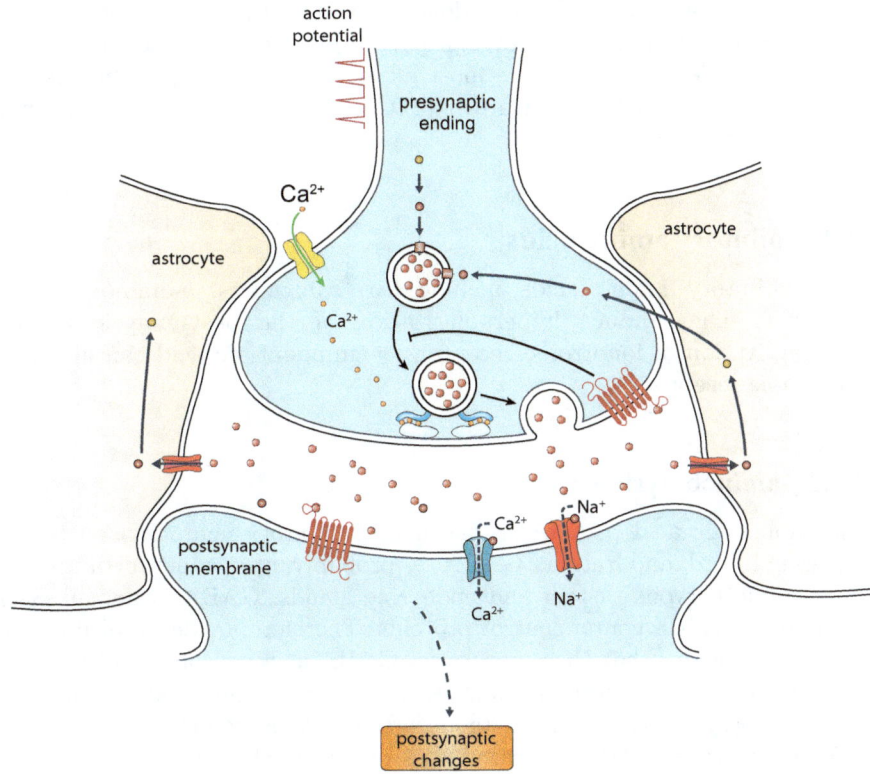

Figure 10.2 Schematic illustration of the processes occurring at the glutamatergic synapse. Glutamate synthesis from glutamine takes place at the presynaptic ending. The arrival of a nerve excitation at the area of the nerve ending causes the opening of voltage-gated channels for Ca^{2+} ions. An increase in the intracytoplasmic concentration of Ca^{2+} ions induces fusion of glutamate-containing vesicles with the presynaptic membrane. The released glutamate diffuses in the synaptic cleft and binds to glutamatergic receptors on the postsynaptic membrane (as well as to receptors on the presynaptic membrane). Activation of ionotropic glutamatergic receptors causes depolarization of the postsynaptic membrane. The action of glutamate is terminated by its uptake by glia cells (modified according to Purves et al., 2008; Popoli et al., 2012).

receptors are made up of several subunits. Four AMPA, five kainate, and six NMDA subunits have been identified, each encoded by a single gene. Metabotropic receptors act through G proteins to increase the intracellular concentration of IP_3 and DAG or decrease the level of intracellular cAMP. Metabotropic glutamate receptors are localized both postsynaptically and presynaptically.

10.2.1.2 Aspartate

Although aspartate is found in the central nervous system and has an excitatory effect on neurons, there is less data on its action as a neurotransmitter compared to glutamate.

Aspartate is synthesized from oxaloacetic acid and glutamate by the enzyme aspartate aminotransferase. However, aspartate has not been shown to be stored in synaptic vesicles. It is therefore most likely released directly from the cytosol of nerve endings. Aspartate activates NMDA receptors, it probably does not act on AMPA receptors.

10.2.2 Inhibitory amino acids

The inhibitory amino acids include two substances, γ-aminobutyric acid and glycine. They induce hyperpolarization of the postsynaptic membrane through activation of ionotropic receptors. γ-aminobutyric acid can also bind to metabotropic receptors.

10.2.2.1 γ-aminobutyric acid

γ-aminobutyric acid (GABA) is the main inhibitory neurotransmitter in the brain, spinal cord and retina. GABA is probably also a neurotransmitter in the autonomic nervous system and endocrine glands. GABA is not an essential metabolite nor is it a component of proteins. Therefore, evidence of its presence in a neuron indicates that the neuron uses GABA as a neurotransmitter.

GABA is synthesized from glutamate by the enzyme glutamate decarboxylase. Detection of the enzyme glutamate decarboxylase is therefore one marker of GABAergic neurons. GABA is located in secretory vesicles, and when released into the synaptic cleft it acts on ionotropic or metabotropic receptors. It increases the passage of Cl^- ions into the neuron, thereby contributing to the hyperpolarization of the postsynaptic membrane. The action of GABA is terminated by both reuptake into neurons and uptake by surrounding glial cells.

In the immature nervous system, GABA binding to GABAergic receptors does not induce hyperpolarization, but instead depolarization. This is due to the fact that immature neurons contain a higher concentration of Cl^- intracellularly compared to the extracellular space. Therefore, the opening of ion channels for Cl^- after occupancy of ionotropic receptors ($GABA_A$ or $GABA_C$) by the neurotransmitter GABA induces Cl^- to pass extraneuronally, thereby depolarizing the neuron. It is only in the mature nervous system that such changes occur in the presence of ion pumps and consequently in the ionic composition of neurons that GABA binding to receptors induces hyperpolarization of the postsynaptic membrane. $GABA_B$ metabotropic receptors are coupled to G protein. Activation of these receptors leads to an increase in conductance for K^+ and an attenuation of adenylate cyclase activity and transport of Ca^{2+} ion extraneuronally, leading to neuronal hyperpolarization.In addition to chemical synapses, some GABAergic neurons in the cerebral cortex also contain electrical synapses. Chemical synapses are formed between the axons of GABAergic neurons and the body of the neurons, while electrical synapses are formed between the dendritic processes of these neurons. Such an arrangement points to the complexity of signal processing in the nervous system.

10.2.2.2 Glycine

Glycine is structurally the simplest amino acid. Involved in many metabolic pathways, it is an essential component of proteins. Glycine is therefore present in all areas of the brain and spinal cord. As an inhibitory neurotransmitter of interneurons, glycine acts predominantly in the brainstem (pons and medulla oblongata) and spinal cord.

The metabolism of glycine in nervous tissue is not precisely characterized. It is not clear whether glycine is synthesized de novo or is taken up by neurons. Glycine is located in secretory vesicles. The released glycine binds to the ionotropic glycine receptor. Occupancy of glycinergic receptors by glycine increases the passage of Cl^- ions into the cell, leading to hyperpolarization of the postsynaptic membrane. In addition to glycinergic receptors, glycine also binds to NMDA receptors, where it acts as a glutamate co-agonist (glycine alone, without glutamate, does not activate NMDA receptors). While glycine binding to the glycinergic receptor induces hyperpolarization, its binding to the NMDA receptor leads to the opposite effect, allowing excitation. As with previous neurotransmitters from the amino acid group, the action of glycine is terminated by both reuptake into neurons and uptake by surrounding glial cells.

As with GABA, glycine can induce excitation instead of inhibition in the immature nervous system. It is thought that some inhibitory synapses may release both glycine and GABA together as neurotransmitters.

10.2.3 Acetylcholine and biogenic amines

Neurons releasing acetylcholine and biogenic amines (norepinephrine, dopamine, epinephrine, serotonin, histamine) share several characteristics. In the brain, they form clusters of cells (but not necessarily compact nuclei), which are mainly located in the brainstem and midbrain. These neurons, although not very numerous, innervate, via long axons that branch abundantly, large subcortical and especially cortical areas of the brain.

Neurons releasing acetylcholine and biogenic amines as neurotransmitters have predominantly modulatory functions in the central nervous system. They act mainly through metabotropic receptors to induce longer lasting changes in postsynaptic membrane permeability, and these changes can persist several times longer than those observed after neurotransmitter binding to ionotropic receptors.

Modulatory neurons are mostly not responsible for fast signal processing, but rather modulate the activity of the nervous system (mainly the cerebral cortex). This modulation is then ultimately responsible for the resulting degree of nervous system reactivity. Modulatory neurons are involved (often indirectly) in information processing. They are of great importance, for example, in the regulation of wakefulness or in emotional reactions.

The release of biogenic amines (but also some other neurotransmitters) in the brain shows some similarity to the release of neurotransmitters in the autonomic nervous system. The axons of autonomic nerves form a network of varicosities in their course in innervated tissue, the so-called *boutons en passant*, from which the neurotransmitter (norepinephrine, acetylcholine) is released into the surroundings.

However, the structure of a classical synapse with presynaptic and postsynaptic membranes is not formed. This mode of neurotransmission is one type of volume transmission. The released neurotransmitter diffuses into the surroundings and can activate a larger number of receptors located on the cells of the innervated tissue. Similarly, as noted above, in the central nervous system, axons (predominantly of aminergic neurons) form boutons en passant-like structures. It is thought that the neurotransmitters released from such structures may influence the activity of a larger number of neurons in their vicinity.

10.2.3.1 Acetylcholine

Acetylcholine is synthesized in the axon terminals from acetyl coenzyme A and choline by the enzyme choline acetyltransferase and is subsequently stored in vesicles. The enzyme choline acetyltransferase is found specifically in the synapses of cholinergic neurons. Its presence is therefore an indicator of cholinergic nerve endings. Choline is transported from the periphery through the bloodstream to the central nervous system, where it serves for the biosynthesis of acetylcholine as well as membrane phospholipids.

Once released into the synaptic cleft, acetylcholine can bind to ionotropic (nicotinic) or metabotropic (muscarinic) receptors located on the postsynaptic membrane. In addition, it can also bind to presynaptically localized autoreceptors (nicotinic, muscarinic), the activation of which reduces the release of acetylcholine from the presynaptic nerve ending. While the action of most small molecule neurotransmitters is terminated by a mechanism of their reuptake into the presynaptic nerve ending, the action of acetylcholine is terminated by its hydrolysis by the synaptically localized enzyme acetylcholinesterase. Choline is reuptaken into the presynaptic termination via a high-affinity choline transporter, and can be used for the resynthesis of acetylcholine.

Acetylcholine is released by neurons as their primary neurotransmitter at almost all levels of the CNS, with approximately 10% of all neurons in the nervous system being cholinergic. Acetylcholine as a neurotransmitter is released at the periphery from:

- motoneurons in neuromuscular junctions;
- preganglionic neurons of the autonomic nervous system;
- postganglionic neurons of the parasympathetic nervous system (as well as some postganglionic neurons of the sympathetic nervous system).

Thus, acetylcholine is the primary neurotransmitter of all neurons that send efferent axons from the CNS to the periphery, both motor and autonomic neurons. Neurons synthesizing acetylcholine as their neurotransmitter form several circumscribed clusters in the brain (Fig. 10.3). Cholinergic neurons are located in the septal and diagonal regions (CH1-3), nucleus basalis Meynerti (CH4), nucleus pedunculopontinus (CH5), and nucleus latero-dorsalis (CH6). In addition, cholinergic neurons are also found in the striatum (nucleus caudatus, putamen) and cerebral cortex.

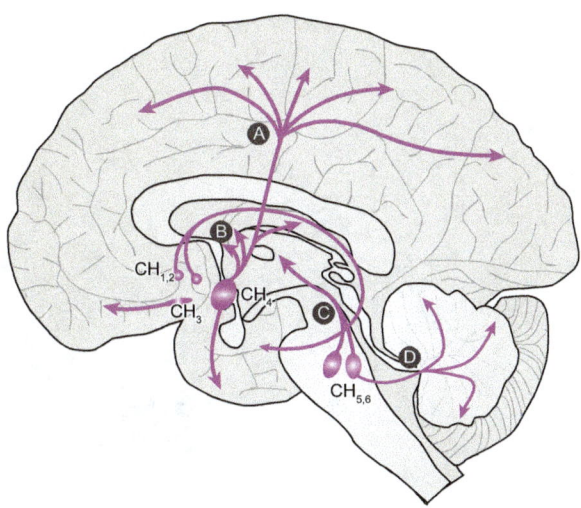

Figure 10.3 Schematic illustration of the localization of major clusters of cholinergic neurons and cholinergic pathways in the brain. CH1-3 - septum and diagonal region, CH4 - ncl. basalis Meynerti, CH5 - ncl. pedunculo-pontinus, CH6 - ncl. latero-dorsalis. A - cholinergic innervation of cortical areas; B - cholinergic pathways in the basal ganglia; C - forebrain innervation emanating from stem cholinergic neurons; D - cholinergic innervation of the cerebellum (modified according to Mravec, 2016).

10.2.3.2 Dopamine

Dopamine is synthesized from the amino acid tyrosine. The biosynthesis of dopamine, the conversion of tyrosine to dyhydroxyphenylalanine (DOPA), catalyzed by the enzyme tyrosine hydroxylase, and the conversion of DOPA to dopamine, catalyzed by the enzyme L-aromatic amino acid decarboxylase, takes place in the cytoplasm of the axon terminal. The synthesized dopamine is subsequently transported by the vesicular transporter for monoamines into secretory vesicles. After depolarization of the nerve ending, dopamine is released from the vesicles into the synaptic cleft. It acts on both postsynaptic and presynaptic dopaminergic metabotropic receptors, which are divided into two major groups, 'D1 -like' and 'D2 -like'. The action of dopamine is terminated by its enzymatic conversion via the extracellularly localized enzyme catechol-O-methyltransferase (COMT), as well as by reuptake via the dopamine transporter, which transports dopamine back to the presynaptic nerve ending. The recaptured dopamine is metabolized by the enzyme monoamine oxidase (MAO), which is located on the membranes of the mitochondria.

Although only about half a million neurons in the human brain synthesize dopamine as their primary neurotransmitter, dopamine is released at almost all levels of the CNS. Dopaminergic neurons are found in areas from the pons to the olfactory bulbus and are designated by the symbols A8 to A16. In the midbrain, they form three clusters (A8, A9, and A10) with an indistinct boundary. A9 dopaminergic neurons are localized in the substantia nigra, predominantly in the pars compacta. Most of the cells of the A10 group are located in the ventral

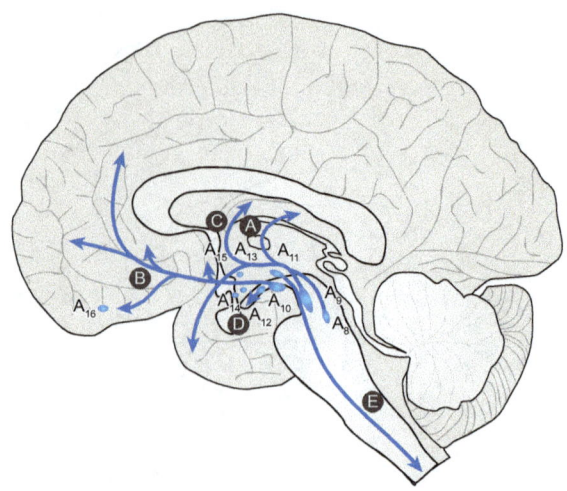

Figure 10.4 Schematic illustration of the localization of dopaminergic neurons and dopaminergic pathways in the brain. A8 - ncl. reticularis pontis oralis, A9 - substantia nigra, pars compacta, A10 - area ventralis tegmenti (Tsai), A11 - ncl. premammillaris dorsalis, A12 - ncl. infundibularis (arcuatus), A13 - zona incerta, A14 - area hypothalamica anterior, A15 - area preoptica, A16 - olfactory bulbus; (A) - nigrostriatal pathway; (B) - mesocortical pathway; (C) - mesolimbic pathway; (D) - tuberoinfundibular pathway; (E) - spinal pathways (modified according to Mravec, 2016).

tegmental area. Neurons of groups A11-A15 are localized in the midbrain. A12-labeled neurons are located in the arcuate nucleus, A16 in the olfactory bulbus. Also, some retinal cells use dopamine as a neurotransmitter (A17). Dopaminergic neurons form several major dopaminergic pathways, which can be divided into ultrashort, intermediate (intermediate), and long based on the length of the axons of the dopaminergic neurons (Fig. 10.4).

10.2.3.3 Norepinephrine

Norepinephrine is synthesized from dopamine found in the cytoplasm by the enzyme dopamine-β-hydroxylase, which is localized on the membrane of secretory vesicles. The norepinephrine released from the vesicles acts in the synaptic cleft on postsynaptic and presynaptic adrenergic receptors, which are divided into two main groups (α and β), the latter being further subdivided into several subtypes. The action of norepinephrine is completed by its enzymatic conversion via the extracellularly localized COMT enzyme as well as by reuptake via the norepinephrine transporter, which transports norepinephrine back to the presynaptic nerve ending. The recaptured norepinephrine is metabolized by the MAO enzyme.

In the brain, noradrenergic neurons are located in the medulla oblongata and the bridge (Fig. 10.5). Noradrenergic A1 neurons are located in the lower part of the medulla oblongata around the nucleus funiculi lateralis and propagate

10. Neurotransmitters and neuromodulators

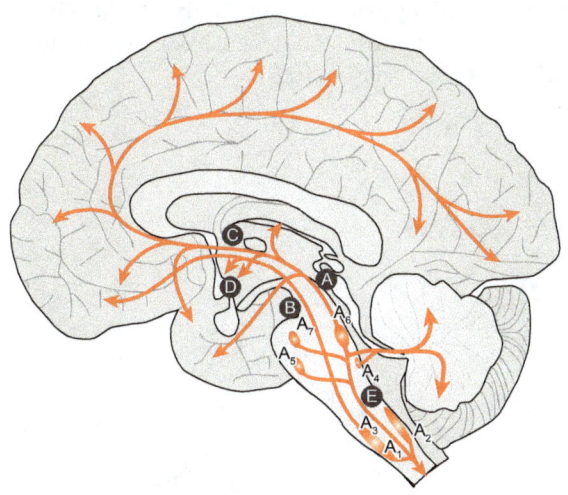

Figure 10.5 Schematic illustration of the localization of noradrenergic neurons and noradrenergic pathways in the brain. A1 - ncl. reticularis lateralis et parvocellularis; A2 - ncl. tractus solitarii; A4 - substantia grisea centralis, pars caudalis; A5 - ncl. reticularis parvocellularis, pars ventralis; A6 - locus coeruleus; A7 - ncl. reticularis parvocellularis; (A) - dorsal noradrenergic bundle; (B) - ventral noradrenergic bundle; (C) – medial bundle in the forebrain; (D) - tractus tegmentalis centralis; (E) - spinal pathways (modified according to Mravec, 2016).

dorsomedially to the lateral part of the reticular formation. A2 group neurons lie in the caudal part of the nucleus tractus solitarii. The A3 group has been demonstrated in rats; its occurrence in the primate brain has not been confirmed. A4 neurons form a subependymal stripe that extends parallel to the fibers of the pedunculus cerebellaris superior and connects with the A6 group at the anterior margin. More than 50% of norepinephrine in the brain is synthesized in cells of the locus coeruleus (A6, LC). Although the LC in humans contains only approximately 12 500 neurons, these provide most of the noradrenergic innervation of the forebrain, brainstem, and spinal cord. A5 neurons are scattered around the nucleus nervi facialis and around the superior olivary complex. A group of A7 neurons is located in the rostral part of the reticular formation in the bridge. Norepinephrine is released at almost all levels of the CNS and in the spinal cord. In the periphery, norepinephrine is synthesized in the adrenal medulla and sympathetic nerve endings.

10.2.3.4 Epinephrine

Epinephrine is synthesized from norepinephrine. Norepinephrine is transported from vesicles into the cytoplasm and converted to epinephrine by the enzyme phenylethanolamine-N-methyltransferase. Subsequently, epinephrine is placed into secretory vesicles. The release, action on receptors and termination of epinephrine action is thought to be similar to that of norepinephrine.

The main source of epinephrine in the body is the chromatin cells of the adrenal medulla. The brain neurons that synthesize epinephrine are localized in the lower part of the brainstem (Fig. 10.6).

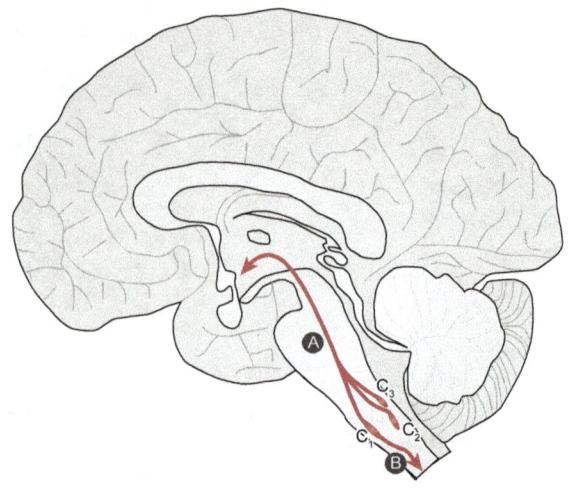

Figure 10.6 Schematic illustration of the localization of adrenergic neurons and adrenergic pathways in the brain. C1 - ncl. reticularis lateralis et parvocellularis; C2 - ncl. tractus solitarii; C3 - ncl. prepositus hypoglossi. A - ascending adrenergic pathways; B - spinal pathways (modified according to Mravec, 2016).

10.2.3.5 Serotonin

Serotonin (5-hydroxytryptamine, 5-HT) is synthesized from the amino acid tryptophan, found in food. In the first step of biosynthesis, 5-hydroxytryptophan is synthetized from tryptophan by the action of the enzyme tryptophan hydroxylase. By the action of the enzyme L-aromatic amino acid decarboxylase, serotonin, which is located in secretory vesicles, is formed from it. The released serotonin acts on both postsynaptic and presynaptic serotoninergic receptors. Its action is terminated by the action of the serotonin transporter, which translocates serotonin back to the presynaptic nerve ending. Serotonin is metabolized by the MAO enzyme. The COMT enzyme is not involved in serotonin metabolism.

10.2.3.6 Histamine

Histamine is synthesized from the amino acid histidine by the enzyme histidine decarboxylase. There are currently four known histaminergic receptors H1 - H4. In the brain, the presence of H1 - H3 receptors has been demonstrated.

Like other biogenic amines, histamine is released at almost all levels of the CNS (Fig. 10.8). In the CNS, histaminergic neurons are located in a circumscribed area of the hypothalamus. In the periphery, mast cells and basophils contain histamine.

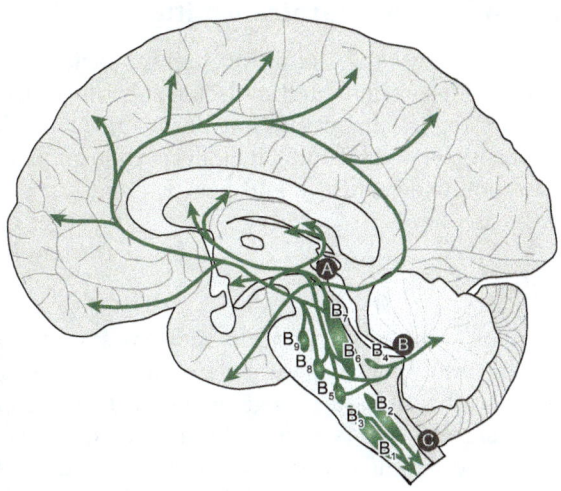

Figure 10.7 Schematic illustration of the localization of serotoninergic neurons and serotoninergic pathways in the brain. B1 - ncl. raphealis pallidus; B2 - ncl. raphealis parvus; B3 - ncl. raphealis magnus; B4 - ncl. raphealis pallidus; B5 - ncl. raphealis pontis; B6 - ncl. raphealis dorsalis; B7 - ncl. raphealis dorsalis; B8 - ncl. linearis caudalis; B9 - ncl. pontis oralis (modified according to Mravec, 2016).

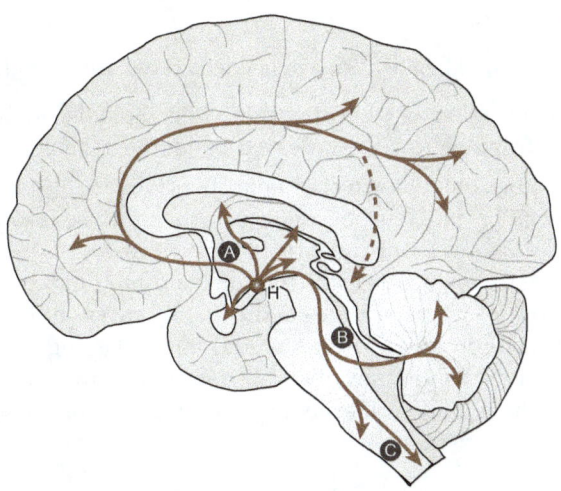

Figure 10.8 Schematic illustration of the localization of histaminergic neurons and histaminergic pathways in the brain. E - ncl. tuberomamillaris; A - ascending pathways innervating the forebrain; B - descending pathways innervating the brainstem and cerebellum; C - spinal pathways (modified according to Mravec, 2016).

10.2.4 Other small molecule neurotransmitters

In addition to excitatory and inhibitory amino acids, acetylcholine, and biogenic amines, neurons use other small molecule substances to transmit signals. This group also includes some chemicals that do not meet all the characteristics of classical neurotransmitters. Examples include carbon monoxide, nitric oxide, hydrogen sulfide, cannabinoids, purines and neurosteroids.

10.3 Neuropeptides

The transmission of signals via peptide molecules is characteristic of the endocrine system. Some neuropeptides were first characterized as hormones of the pituitary gland and peripheral tissues (e.g. in the gastrointestinal tract). Later, many peptides were shown to meet the characteristics of neurotransmitters. Currently, more than 50 different neuropeptides are known.

Peptide neurotransmitters meet several (some all) of the criteria necessary for their classification as neurotransmitters. However, there are differences in the biosynthesis and release of peptide neurotransmitters compared to small molecule neurotransmitters. Characteristics of peptide neurotransmitters include:

- are synthesized in the body of the neuron, where the necessary synthetic apparatus is located (small molecule neurotransmitters are synthesized in the nerve ending);
- a single gene may encode several types of neuropeptides; these arise from different enzymatic processing of the product of that gene (e.g. neuropeptides of the proopiomelanocortin group);
- are present in tissues in much lower concentrations compared to classical neurotransmitters;
- a higher frequency of excitations is needed to release them from the neurons;
- enzymatic conversion of neuropeptides (e.g. opioids, tachykinins, CGRP) can produce fragments with preserved or modified biological activity.

More recent findings have shown that neuropeptides are also frequently released from dendrites in the brain. Neuropeptides can then diffuse into the surroundings and act on neurons distant from the site of their release.

Neuropeptides act as neurotransmitters or neuromodulators in various neural circuits. The washout of neuropeptides and the occupation of their receptors does not usually result in rapid but rather slow and longer lasting changes in neuronal excitability and activity. This may also be manifested by a change in neuronal gene expression, which may underlie long-term morphological and functional changes in the nervous system.

Group	Neuropeptide
Neurohypophyseal hormones	vasopressin oxytocin
Hypothalamic releasing hormones	corticoliberin urocortin-1, -2, -3 urotensin-II sauvagine thyreoliberin somatostatin
POMC derivatives	adrenocorticotropic hormone α-, β-, γ-melanocyte-stimulating hormone β-endorphin enkephalin dynorphin
Tachykinins	substance P neurokinin A neurokinin B neuropeptide K neuropeptide γ
Neuropeptides of the secretin-VIP-glucagon family	glucagon-like peptide-1 vasoactive intestinal polypeptide histidine isoleucine peptide pituitary adenylate cyclase activating peptide
Other neuropeptides	5-HT modulin adrenomedullin agouti related protein amylin angiotensin II apelin brain natriuretic peptide calcitonin gene-related peptide cocaine- and amphetamine-regulated transcript endomorphin 1, 2 galanin galanin-like peptide ghrelin cholecystokinin chromogranin A, B, secretoneurin melanin-concentrating hormone neuropeptide AF neuropeptide B neuropeptide EI neuropeptide FF neuropeptide GE neuropeptide S neuropeptide SF neuropeptide tyrosine neuropeptide W neurotensin nociceptin/orphanin FQ nocistatin orexin/hypocretin prolactin-releasing peptide

Table 10.2 Overview of the groups of large molecule neurotransmitters or neuromodulators (modified according to von Bohlen-Halbach and Dermietzel, 2006).

11

Electrical synapses

Electrical synapses are relatively rarely represented in the mammalian nervous system. Through these synapses, the cytoplasm of two neurons is seamlessly connected via bridging channels with a diameter of 1.5 nm (Fig. 11.1). These junctions or channels (connexons) are formed by the proteins of the two neurons forming an electrical synapse or "gap junction", thereby electrically connecting the neurons. The bridging junction allows a direct flow of ions between the neurons, while the electrical synapses are characterized electrophysiologically by low resistance. No neurotransmitter is released at these synapses. The synaptic delay is extremely short, since the electrical activity spreads very rapidly from one neuron to another. Because electrical synapses are largely not highly modulatable, they are not involved in the regulation of more complex functions, as is the case with chemical synapses. However, they are found in those circuits where precise synchronization of neuronal activity is required, for example, in circuits involved in rapid saccadic eye movements. In the effector organs, electrical synapses ensure the transmission of excitations between the smooth muscle cells of the digestive tube (nexus), which provide peristaltic movements, and between cardiomyocytes (intercalary discs), where they ensure the synchronization of contractions.

Because current can flow through tight junctions in either direction, it is difficult to determine which membrane is presynaptic and which is postsynaptic, especially if the electrical synapse is formed between two dendrites, two neuronal bodies, or two axons. However, there are probably also electrical synapses where the transfer of ions (and hence signals) occurs in only one direction.

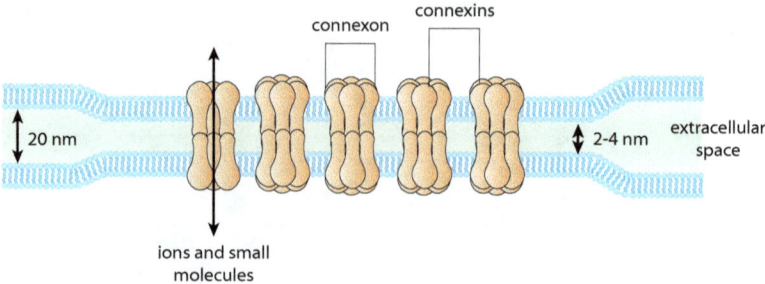

Figure 11.1 Schematic illustration of an electrical synapse. The membranes of two neurons are connected to each other by gap junctions, which are formed by two connected connexons, called half channels. Each connexon consists of six subunits, the connexins. A connexon in the membrane of one cell connects to another connexon located in the membrane of an adjacent cell. This creates a channel through which ions and small molecules can pass without entering the extracellular space. Connexons have a closed channel lumen at rest. When a neuron is activated, a conformational change of the connexons occurs, resulting in the opening of the channel lumen through which ions can pass from one neuron to another. The direct transfer of ions allows very rapid transmission of signals across electrical synapses (modified according to Purves et al., 2008; Bloomfield and Volgyi, 2009).

Part V. Processing of signals in the nervous system

Processing of signals in the nervous system takes place at several levels, with the primary function played by processes occurring at the level of synapses, whose structure and function are determined by genetic factors. The accumulation of several synapses interacting with each other to form microcircuits, which are micrometer in size and process signals at millisecond intervals. The microcircuits are grouped into dendritic subunits, with the dendritic branching of a single neuron providing the basis for the integrative activity of the neuron. A single neuron typically contains several dendritic branching points, which increases the level of signal processing complexity in the nervous system. Interactions between neurons located in a particular area give rise to local circuits that perform signal processing characteristic of that area of the nervous system. Circuits connecting multiple areas represent a higher level of signal processing that results in organism-specific behavior.

12

Neuron as integrator

Each neuron represents a signal integrator. In sensory and sensory neurons, the integration of signals induced by the action of stimuli specific to the sensory or sensory neuron occurs. Other neurons integrate signals that act on them mainly in the form of neurotransmitter molecules that bind to receptors present on dendrites and the cell body. Some receptive areas of the dendrite and cell body membrane are part of excitatory synapses, others inhibitory. At any given time, hundreds to thousands of signals may act on a single neuron through excitatory and inhibitory synapses. At the same time, most neurons are almost constantly under the influence of a multitude of excitatory and inhibitory signals, and the neuron responds to these stimuli with a particular response. If the EPSP summation exceeds the IPSP summation and the initiating segment of the axon is sufficiently activated, an action potential is generated. However, if the resulting summation does not reach the threshold required for action potential formation, the axon does not transmit any neural excitations. Thus, each dendrite-cell body complex represents a miniature integration center that conditions the generation of action potentials depending on the total excitatory and inhibitory activity of the neuron's receptive membrane. The axon subsequently provides the encoding of signals into the form of action potentials and the transmission of these signals to other neurons or effector cells (e.g., myocytes, glandular cells).

Each postsynaptic membrane of a neuron and effector cell contains hundreds to thousands of receptors. Each of these receptor's function as a specialized decoder that responds to a given stimulus with a specific response. Examples are the excitatory action of acetylcholine via the nicotinic receptors of the neuromuscular disc (contraction of skeletal muscle) and the inhibitory action via muscarinic receptors in cardiac tissue (slowing of the heart rate).

12.1 Functions of dendrites

The function of dendrites is partly expressed by their characteristic morphological differences in different regions of the brain and spinal cord. The diversity of dendrite morphology is determined by their branching pattern and the richness of branching and the different variations in the morphology of their spinous processes. Dendritic spines, whose volume is usually less than 1 µm^3 show diversity in shape and size. Dendritic spines, meanwhile, exhibit a high degree of plasticity, and can form, disappear, renew, and change their size and shape rapidly, depending on a range of factors. The morphological and functional properties of dendrites are the result of both genetic and epigenetic factors (external environmental factors). For example, the size of the spine head is directly proportional to the number of postsynaptic receptors and the number of anchored synaptic vesicles in the presynaptic nerve ending.

Dendritic spines contain postsynaptic dense formations that are attached to the inner surface of the postsynaptic membrane. They are composed of a large number of signaling proteins whose role is to regulate the strength of synaptic connections, modify the morphology of spine processes, and influence the synthesis of synapse-specific proteins. Scaffolding proteins in the region of postsynaptic densities provide the link between the stimulus acting on membrane glutamatergic receptors with receptors on the smooth endoplasmic reticulum, with receptors on actin filaments of the cytoskeleton, and with morphogens that influence the shape and size of spines. Each spinous process contains a dense network of actin filaments, referred to as the spinous apparatus, which serves:

- as a support and skeleton anchoring functional molecules;
- as a means of moving substances from the dendrite to the postsynaptic density;
- for the mobility of the spines;
- as a source of morphogens that influence synaptic function during development and plasticity.

In dendrites, DNA translation takes place, with mRNA molecules attached to ribosomes being transported into dendrites up to near the base of the spines. Molecular triggers activate the mRNA located in the spines, resulting in the synthesis of synapse-specific proteins there. The synthesis of proteins directly at the synapse region thus allows an active feedback effect on DNA transcription in the nucleus of the neuron. The degree of activity of a given synapse thus influences mRNA production, transport of ribosomes by microtubules, and acts selectively on certain ribosomes that are translocated to the vicinity of a given spine protrusion, where translation of mRNA into proteins required in that spine subsequently occurs. Thus, in neurons, unlike most cells, translation of mRNA occurs not only in the cell body but also in the dendrites, which is essential for the processes associated with the specialization of individual synapses. The presence of factors required for translation and the presence of mRNA allows individual synapses to independently regulate the strength of synaptic connections through local protein synthesis.

It is estimated that of the 10^{14} synapses that are found on about 10^{11} neurons in the human cerebral cortex, more than 90% are made up of excitatory axodendritic synapses. Excitatory glutamatergic receptors are found primarily on dendritic spines, and inhibitory GABAergic receptors are found on dendrites predominantly outside the spines, on cell bodies and axon initial segments. Synaptic activity of dendrites is an important factor in the biochemical mechanisms regulating synapse-specific protein synthesis. Several of these proteins are likely to be involved in phenomena such as learning and memory. Signal processing conditioned by stimulation of ionotropic receptors of neurotransmitter systems and metabotropic receptors of modulatory systems further increases the degree of complexity compared to the simple summation of EPSP and IPSP underlying action potential generation.

12.2 Spontaneous neuronal activity

Some neurons generate action potentials only when they are sufficiently depolarized by stimuli applied to their receptive field, and for sensory and sensory neurons the stimuli may be different modalities (e.g., mechanical force, temperature, photons). For interneurons and motor neurons, it is excitatory neurotransmitters released by synapses on the dendrites and bodies of these neurons.

But there are also neurons that show spontaneous activation, the extent of which is modulated by synaptic inputs. Spontaneously active neurons contain intrinsic mechanisms that lead to spontaneous depolarization that is sufficient to elicit the generation of an action potential. The synaptic influences on these neurons are the same as on other neurons (summation of EPSP and IPSP), but the activity of spontaneously active neurons can also be modulated by other, non-synaptic factors, such as circulating hormones. Neurons with spontaneous (intrinsic) activity provide specific functions that include, for example, circadian rhythms and hormone secretion.

13

Processing of signal in neural circuits

After signals are generated in sensory or sensory endings or in other structures of the nervous system (e.g., endogenous signal generation in the brain), the signals are transmitted to the central nervous system and, after their processing, regulatory signals are formed that modulate the activity of other neurons or effector cells involved in neuronal circuits. Neuronal circuits are a series of interconnected neurons that are linked together in various ways.

13.1 Excitatory neuronal circuits

In excitatory neuronal circuits, neurons are connected via excitatory synapses. An example is a neuronal pathway that begins at a specialized voltage-gated receptor in a muscle spindle. Afferent fibers from the muscle spindle form an excitatory synapse with the motoneuron. The sensory neuron, the motoneuron, and the muscle they innervate thus form a simple neural circuit in which two excitatory synapses are present.

In excitatory neuronal circuits, excitation can be transferred from one neuron to another neuron, from multiple neurons to one neuron (convergence), and from one neuron to multiple other neurons (divergence) (Fig. 13.1).

13.2 The importance of inhibition

Inhibition is as important a neuronal process as excitation. Inhibitory neurons and the neural circuits of which they are a part, regulate the activity of excitatory neurons and excitatory neural circuits so that these are not overactive and so that neurons are not eventually damaged by overexcitation. Inhibitory circuits significantly affect the processing of sensory and sensory stimuli, an example being lateral inhibition, which allows for increased sensory discrimination (Fig. 13.1) .

13.2.1 Presynaptic inhibition and presynaptic facilitation

Presynaptic inhibition is a process that occurs when one neuron exerts an inhibitory action via a neurotransmitter released at an axo-axonal synapse located near the axon terminal of another neuron (Fig. 13.1). The result is a reduced release of excitatory neurotransmitter from the presynaptic ending of this second neuron. That process involves changes in the permeability of ion channels for Cl^-, K^+, and Ca^{2+}. The release of inhibitory neurotransmitter by the neuron at the axo-axonal synapse causes the opening of channels for Cl^- and K^+ ions at the termination of the second neuron. Consequently, there is a decrease in Ca^{2+} ion entry into this neuron via voltage-gated channels. The decreased Ca^{2+} ion influx causes a decrease in excitatory neurotransmitter release from the neuron's terminus at the synapse that this neuron forms with the other neuron.

Presynaptic facilitation (presynaptic excitation) is the process that occurs when a given neuron exerts excitatory influence through the release of an excitatory neurotransmitter at the axo-axonal synapse it forms at the axon terminal of another neuron (Fig. 13.1). Presynaptic release of the neurotransmitter causes closure of the K^+ channels, resulting in prolonged action potential duration as the repolarization phase is slowed. This causes an increase in the entry of Ca^{2+} ions into the axon termination of the neuron, which increases the release of excitatory neurotransmitter from its synaptic termination, which it forms with the next neuron.

Presynaptic inhibition and facilitation represents an important process involved in signal processing in the central nervous system. These processes allow the transmission of signals between two neurons to be selectively influenced without directly affecting the reactivity of the innervated neuron, which can therefore respond to signals transmitted at other synapses.

13.2.2 Feedback inhibition

A neuron can regulate its own activity or that of other neurons in its surroundings by feedback (recurrent) inhibition (Fig. 13.1). In this case, a single collateral neuron extending from the axon innervates an inhibitory interneuron, which in turn inhibits the activity of that neuron. Recurrent inhibition can also be mediated by reciprocal dendro-dendritic synapses. This type of synapse is found in various brain regions, such as the olfactory bulbus, posterior horns of the spinal cord, retina, thalamus, and suprachiasmatic nucleus.

13.2.3 Forward inhibition

In forward inhibition, the activity of one or more neurons inhibits another neuron or group of neurons (Fig. 13.1). The feedforward inhibitory circuit is characterized by the presence of one or more inhibitory interneurons in this circuit. These interneurons mediate influence in the forward direction to more distal regions of a given pathway. Forward inhibition is used, for example, in the processing of sensory or sensory signals. Here, it may also be involved in contrast enhancement, also via lateral inhibition.

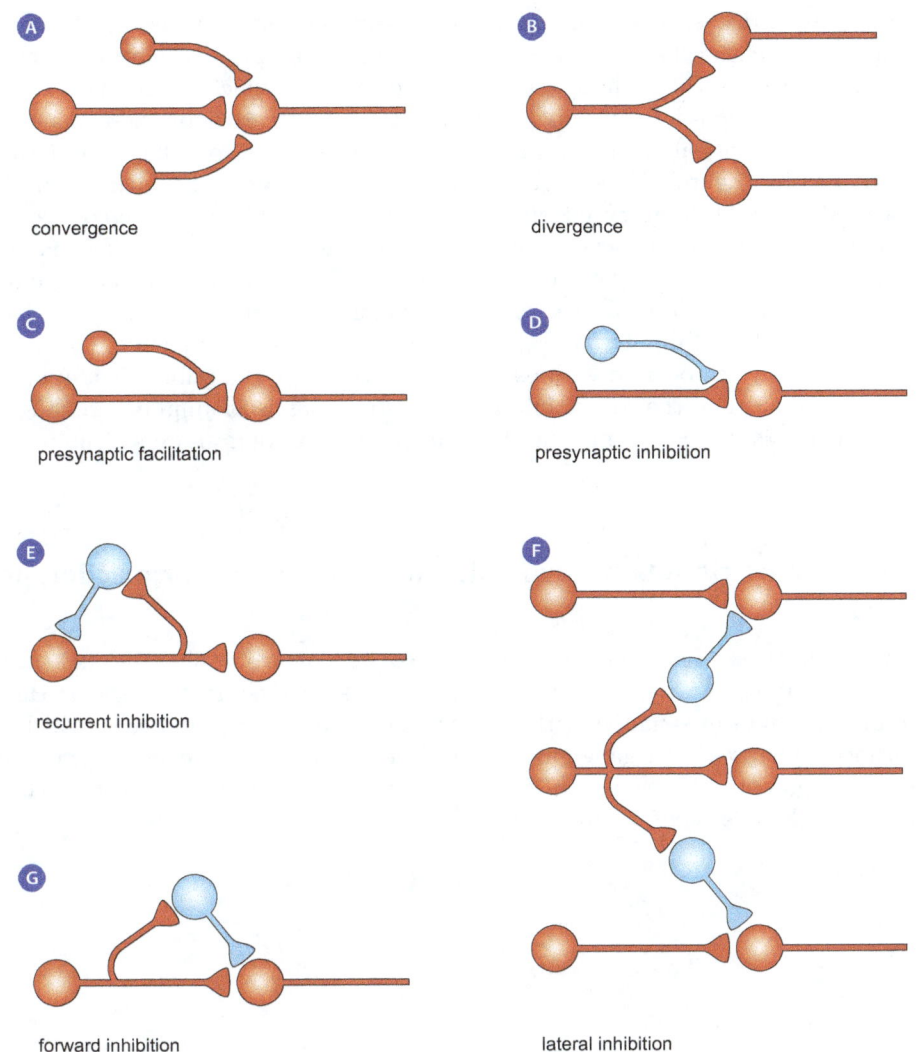

Figure 13.1 Schematic illustration of signal processing mechanisms in the nervous system. Excitatory neurons are shown in red, inhibitory neurons in blue (modified according to Schmidt, 1976; Bailey et al., 2000; Hall, 2020).

Forward inhibition is also used in the action of muscle spindles in the stretch reflex. Afferent fibers from neuromuscular spindles excite inhibitory interneurons, which act inhibitory on α-motoneurons innervating skeletal muscles.

13.2.4 Lateral inhibition

Lateral inhibition (lateral attenuation) is one of the basic signal processing mechanisms in the nervous system. This physiological mechanism is used, for example, by all sensory systems in the processing of nerve signals. An example is the discrimination between two stimuli acting on receptive structures in close proximity. Two neural pathways are activated, each of which transmits a signal produced in response to one of the acting stimuli. In each of these neuronal pathways, the signaling is amplified and the activity of the surrounding interconnecting neurons is suppressed in order to preserve the identity of the applied stimulus. Inhibitory interneurons interact with adjacent interconnecting neurons, resulting in an increase in the signal-to-noise ratio. This effect is also referred to as the targeting or sharpening effect. Thus, for example, background noise generated by blood flow through the inner ear is not normally perceived because it is filtered out by lateral inhibition in the auditory pathway, and the neuronal activity associated with exposure to relevant sound stimuli is amplified. In the visual system, the role of inhibitory interneurons is to amplify signaling so that contrast is increased, making boundaries and contours more salient to the observer.

13.3 Neuronal circuits involving neurons that do not form action potentials

There are also neuronal circuits that contain neurons that do not form action potentials. Examples are neuronal circuits located in the retina. Here, photoreceptors form synapses with bipolar neurons and horizontal cells, which in turn form synapses with ganglion cells. Neither of these neuron types generates an action potential. However, a graded response is present nonetheless, which modulates the release of neurotransmitters also in a graded fashion.

List of abbreviations

5-HT	5-hydroxytryptamine (serotonin)
AC	adenylate cyclase
AM	amplitude modulation
AMPA R	an ionotropic type of receptor for glutamate (the agonist is γ-amino-3-hydroxy-5-methyl-4-isoxazolepropionic acid)
ATP	adenosine triphosphate
BDNF	brain growth factor
CaM	calmodulin
CaMKIV	calmodulin-dependent kinase IV
cAMP	cyclic adenosine monophosphate
CNS	central nervous system
COMT	catechol-O-methyltransferase
CREB	cAMP-responsive element
CRH	corticoliberin
DNA	deoxyribonucleic acid
DOPA	3,4-dihydroxyphenylalanine
EPSP	excitatory postsynaptic potential
FM	frequency modulation
GABA	γ-aminobutyric acid
GluR1	subunit of the glutamate receptor
IPSP	inhibitory postsynaptic potential
MAO	monoamine oxidase
mRNA	mediator RNA
mtDNA	mitochondrial DNA
NMDA	ionotropic subtype of the glutamate receptor (the agonist is N-methyl-d-aspartate)
PKA	protein kinase A
PNS	peripheral nervous system
RNA	ribonucleic acid
rRNA	ribosomal RNA
TH	tyrosine hydroxylase
tRNA	transfer RNA

References

Abbott NJ, Ronnback L, Hansson E. Astrocyte-endothelial interactions at the blood-brain barrier. Nat Rev Neurosci 2006; 7: 41-53.

Ables JL, Breunig JJ, Eisch AJ, Rakic P. Not(ch) just development: Notch signalling in the adult brain. Nat Rev Neurosci 2011; 12: 269-83.

Agnati LF, Zoli M, Stromberg I, Fuxe K. Intercellular communication in the brain: wiring versus volume transmission. Neuroscience 1995; 69: 711-26.

Amaral P, Carbonell-Sala S, De La Vega FM, Faial T, Frankish A, Gingeras T, Guigo R, Harrow JL, Hatzigeorgiou AG, Johnson R, Murphy TD, Pertea M, Pruitt KD, Pujar S, Takahashi H, Ulitsky I, Varabyou A, Wells CA, Yandell M, Carninci P, Salzberg SL. The status of the human gene catalogue. Nature 2023; 622: 41-7.

Aragon C, Lopez-Corcuera B. Structure, function and regulation of glycine neurotransporters. Eur J Pharmacol 2003; 479: 249-62.

Azevedo FA, Carvalho LR, Grinberg LT, Farfel JM, Ferretti RE, Leite RE, Jacob Filho W, Lent R, Herculano-Houzel S. Equal numbers of neuronal and non-neuronal cells make the human brain an isometrically scaled-up primate brain. J Comp Neurol 2009; 513: 532-41.

Badiani A, Belin D, Epstein D, Calu D, Shaham Y. Opiate versus psychostimulant addiction: the differences do matter. Nat Rev Neurosci 2011; 12: 685-700.

Bailey CH, Giustetto M, Huang YY, Hawkins RD, Kandel ER. Is heterosynaptic modulation essential for stabilizing Hebbian plasticity and memory? Nat Rev Neurosci 2000; 1: 11-20.

Barrett KE, Barman SM, Brooks HL, Yuan JXJ. Ganong's Review of Medical Physiology, 26e. New York, NY: McGraw-Hill Education, 2019, pp.

Bean BP. The action potential in mammalian central neurons. Nat Rev Neurosci 2007; 8: 451-65.

Bear MF, Connors BW, Paradiso MA. Neuroscience: exploring the brain. Baltimore: Lippincott Williams & Wilkins, 2015, 975 pp.

Bloomfield SA, Volgyi B. The diverse functional roles and regulation of neuronal gap junctions in the retina. Nat Rev Neurosci 2009; 10: 495-506.

Boehning D, Snyder SH. Novel neural modulators. Annu Rev Neurosci 2003; 26: 105-31.

Brady ST, Siegel GJ, Albers RW, Price DL. Basic neurochemistry: Molecular, cellular, and medical aspects. San Diego: Elsevier Academic Press, 2005, 1016 pp.

Brodal P. Central nervous system: structure and function. Martin: Osveta, 2008, 517 pp.

Carlezon WA, Jr., Duman RS, Nestler EJ. The many faces of CREB. Trends Neurosci 2005; 28: 436-45.

Caulfield MP, Birdsall NJ. International Union of Pharmacology. XVII. Classification of muscarinic acetylcholine receptors. Pharmacol Rev 1998; 50: 279-90.

Civantos Calzada B, Aleixandre de Artinano A. Alpha-adrenoceptor subtypes. Pharmacol Res 2001; 44: 195-208.

Coleman M. Axon degeneration mechanisms: commonality amid diversity. Nat Rev Neurosci 2005; 6: 889-98.

Crosnier C, Stamataki D, Lewis J. Organizing cell renewal in the intestine: stem cells, signals and combinatorial control. Nat Rev Genet 2006; 7: 349-59.

Danbolt NC. Glutamate uptake. Prog Neurobiol 2001; 65: 1-105.

Dingledine R, Borges K, Bowie D, Traynelis SF. The glutamate receptor ion channels. Pharmacol Rev 1999; 51: 7-61.

Feder A, Nestler EJ, Charney DS. Psychobiology and molecular genetics of resilience. Nat Rev Neurosci 2009; 10: 446-57.

Fields RD. The other brain. New York: Simon & Schuster, 2009, 371 pp.

Flatmark T. Catecholamine biosynthesis and physiological regulation in neuroendocrine cells. Acta Physiol Scand 2000; 168: 1-17.

Fujita T. Present status of paraneuron concept. Arch Histol Cytol 1989; 52 Suppl: 1-8.

Fukuda T, Kosaka T. The dual network of GABAergic interneurons linked by both chemical and electrical synapses: a possible infrastructure of the cerebral cortex. Neurosci Res 2000; 38: 123-30.

Gadea A, Lopez-Colome AM. Glial transporters for glutamate, glycine, and GABA III. Glycine transporters. J Neurosci Res 2001a; 64: 218-22.

Gadea A, Lopez-Colome AM. Glial transporters for glutamate, glycine, and GABA: II. GABA transporters. J Neurosci Res 2001b; 63: 461-8.

Gladkevich A, Korf J, Hakobyan VP, Melkonyan KV. The peripheral GABAergic system as a target in endocrine disorders. Auton Neurosci 2006; 124: 1-8.

Govindarajan A, Kelleher RJ, Tonegawa S. A clustered plasticity model of long-term memory engrams. Nat Rev Neurosci 2006; 7: 575-83.

Gu Q. Neuromodulatory transmitter systems in the cortex and their role in cortical plasticity. Neuroscience 2002; 111: 815-35.

Hall J. Guyton and Hall Textbook of Medical Physiology. Philadelphia: Elsevier, 2020, pp.

Hallberg M, Nyberg F. Neuropeptide conversion to bioactive fragments--an important pathway in neuromodulation. Curr Protein Pept Sci 2003; 4: 31-44.

Hammer GD, McPhee SJ. Pathophysiology of Disease: An Introduction to Clinical Medicine. New York: McGraw-Hill Medical, 2018, 835 pp.

Hein L, Kobilka BK. Adrenergic receptor signal transduction and regulation. Neuropharmacology 1995; 34: 357-66.

Hill SJ, Ganellin CR, Timmerman H, Schwartz JC, Shankley NP, Young JM, Schunack W, Levi R, Haas HL. International Union of Pharmacology. XIII. Classification of histamine receptors. Pharmacol Rev 1997; 49: 253-78.

Jacobson S, Pugsley S, Marcus EM. Neuroanatomy for the neuroscientist. New York: Springer, 2025, 950 pp.

Kandel ER, Koester JD, Mack SH, Siegelbaum SA. Principles of neural science. New York: McGraw-Hill Medical, 2021, 1696 pp.

Kiernan JA, Rajakumar R. Barr's The Human Nervous System. Baltimore: Lippincott Williams & Wilkins, 2013, 448 pp.

Kirstein SL, Insel PA. Autonomic nervous system pharmacogenomics: a progress report. Pharmacol Rev 2004; 56: 31-52.

Langer SZ. 25 years since the discovery of presynaptic receptors: present knowledge and future perspectives. Trends Pharmacol Sci 1997; 18: 95-9.

Legendre P. The glycinergic inhibitory synapse. Cell Mol Life Sci 2001; 58: 760-93.

Loffelholz K. Brain choline has a typical precursor profile. J Physiol Paris 1998; 92: 235-9.

Ludwig M, Leng G. Dendritic peptide release and peptide-dependent behaviours. Nat Rev Neurosci 2006; 7: 126-36.

Lukas RJ, Changeux JP, Le Novere N, Albuquerque EX, Balfour DJ, Berg DK, Bertrand D, Chiappinelli VA, Clarke PB, Collins AC, Dani JA, Grady SR, Kellar KJ, Lindstrom JM, Marks MJ, Quik M, Taylor PW, Wonnacott S. International Union of Pharmacology. XX. Current status of the nomenclature for nicotinic acetylcholine receptors and their subunits. Pharmacol Rev 1999; 51: 397-401.

Matthews G, Fuchs P. The diverse roles of ribbon synapses in sensory neurotransmission. Nat Rev Neurosci 2010; 11: 812-22.

Mei L, Xiong WC. Neuregulin 1 in neural development, synaptic plasticity and schizophrenia. Nat Rev Neurosci 2008; 9: 437-52.

Mombaerts P. Genes and ligands for odorant, vomeronasal and taste receptors. Nat Rev Neurosci 2004; 5: 263-78.

Morris JF, Ludwig M. Magnocellular dendrites: prototypic receiver/transmitters. J Neuroendocrinol 2004; 16: 403-8.

Mravec B. 7. Basic neurophysiology of the central nervous system (in relation to the mechanism of action of psychopharmaceuticals). In: Pečeňák J, Kořínková V, eds. Psychopharmacology. Bratislava: Wolters Kluwer 2016; 69-105.

Muchowski PJ, Wacker JL. Modulation of neurodegeneration by molecular chaperones. Nat Rev Neurosci 2005; 6: 11-22.

Noback CR, Strominger NL, Demarest RJ, Ruggiero DA. The human nervous system. Structure and function. New Jersey: Humana Press, 2005, 477 pp.

Nolte J. Elsevier's Integrated Neuroscience. Philadelphia: Mosby Elsevier, 2007, 245 pp.

Okuda T, Haga T. High-affinity choline transporter. Neurochem Res 2003; 28: 483-8.

Owens DF, Kriegstein AR. Is there more to GABA than synaptic inhibition? Nat Rev Neurosci 2002; 3: 715-27.

Parsons ME, Ganellin CR. Histamine and its receptors. Br J Pharmacol 2006; 147 Suppl 1: S127-35.

Paterson D, Nordberg A. Neuronal nicotinic receptors in the human brain. Prog Neurobiol 2000; 61: 75-111.

Petrovický P. Anatomy with topography and clinical applications. Volume III. Neuroanatomy, sensory organs and skin. Martin: Osveta, 2002, 542 pp.

Popoli M, Yan Z, McEwen BS, Sanacora G. The stressed synapse: the impact of stress and glucocorticoids on glutamate transmission. Nat Rev Neurosci 2012; 13: 22-37.

Purves D, Augustine GJ, Fitzpatrick D, Hall WC, LaMantia AS, Mooney RD, Platt ML, White L. Neuroscience. Sunderland Sinauer Associated 2017, 960 pp.

Rehfeld JF. The new biology of gastrointestinal hormones. Physiol Rev 1998; 78: 1087-108.

Ribak CE, Roberts RC. GABAergic synapses in the brain identified with antisera to GABA and its synthesizing enzyme, glutamate decarboxylase. J Electron Microsc Tech 1990; 15: 34-48.

Ribrault C, Sekimoto K, Triller A. From the stochasticity of molecular processes to the variability of synaptic transmission. Nat Rev Neurosci 2011; 12: 375-87.

Sarter M, Parikh V. Choline transporters, cholinergic transmission and cognition. Nat Rev Neurosci 2005; 6: 48-56.

Shepherd GM. Synaptic organization of the brain. New York: Oxford University Press, 2004, 719 pp.

Schmidt RF. Fundamentals of neurophysiology. New York: Springer-Verlag, 1976, 293 pp.

Snyder SH, Ferris CD. Novel neurotransmitters and their neuropsychiatric relevance. Am J Psychiatry 2000; 157: 1738-51.

Squire L, Berg D, Bloom F, Du Lac S, Ghosh A, Spitzer N. Fundamental neuroscience. San Diego: Academic Press, 2012, 1152 pp.

Stein LD. End of the beginning. Nature 2012: 915-6.

Steward O. Functional neuroscience. New York: Springer-Verlag, 2000, 549 pp.

Sykova E. Extrasynaptic volume transmission and diffusion parameters of the extracellular space. Neuroscience 2004; 129: 861-76.

Vizi ES. Role of high-affinity receptors and membrane transporters in nonsynaptic communication and drug action in the central nervous system. Pharmacol Rev 2000; 52: 63-89.

Vizi ES, Kiss JP, Lendvai B. Nonsynaptic communication in the central nervous system. Neurochem Int 2004; 45: 443-51.

Volpicelli LA, Levey AI. Muscarinic acetylcholine receptor subtypes in cerebral cortex and hippocampus. Prog Brain Res 2004; 145: 59-66.

von Bohlen-Halbach O, Dermietzel R. Neurotransmitters and neuromodulators: handbook of receptors and biological effects. Weinheim: Wiley-VCH, 2006, 386 pp.

Webster RA. Neurotransmitters, drugs and brain function. Chichester: John Wiley & Sons, 2001, 534 pp.

West AE, Griffith EC, Greenberg ME. Regulation of transcription factors by neuronal activity. Nat Rev Neurosci 2002; 3: 921-31.

www.ingramcontent.com/pod-product-compliance
Lightning Source LLC
Chambersburg PA
CBHW050324230526
45471CB00005B/2335